The Restoration of Teeth

T. R. Pitt Ford
PhD, BDS Lond., FDS, RCPS
Senior Lecturer
Department of Conservative Dental Surgery
United Medical and Dental Schools
Guy's Hospital, London SE1

SECOND EDITION

OXFORD

BLACKWELL SCIENTIFIC PUBLICATIONS

LONDON EDINBURGH BOSTON
MELBOURNE PARIS BERLIN VIENNA

© 1985, 1992 by
Blackwell Scientific Publications
Editorial Offices:
Osney Mead, Oxford OX2 0EL
25 John Street, London WC1N 2BL
23 Ainslie Place, Edinburgh EH3 6AJ
3 Cambridge Center, Cambridge
    Massachusetts 02142, USA
54 University Street, Carlton
    Victoria 3053, Australia

Other Editorial Offices:
Arnette SA
2, rue Casimir-Delavigne
75006 Paris
France

Blackwell Wissenschaft
Meinekestrasse 4
D-1000 Berlin 15
Germany

Blackwell MZV
Feldgasse 13
A-1238 Wien
Austria

First published 1985
Second edition 1992

Set by Excel Typesetters, Hong Kong
Printed and bound in Great Britain by
The Alden Press

DISTRIBUTORS

Marston Book Services Ltd
PO Box 87
Oxford OX2 0DT
(*Orders*: Tel: 0865 791155
            Fax: 0865 791927
            Telex: 837515)

USA
Blackwell Scientific Publications, Inc.
3 Cambridge Center
Cambridge, MA 02142
(*Orders*: Tel: 800 759-6102)

Canada
Times Mirror Professional Publishing, Ltd.
5240 Finch Avenue East
Scarborough, Ontario M1S 5A2
(*Orders*: Tel: 416 298-1588)

Australia
Blackwell Scientific Publications
(Australia) Pty Ltd
54 University Street
Carlton, Victoria 3053
(*Orders*: Tel: 03 347-0300)

British Library
Cataloguing in Publication Data

Pitt Ford, T. R.
    The restoration of teeth. — 2nd ed.
    1. Dentistry
    I. Title
    617.6

    ISBN 0-632-03252-9

Contents

Preface to the second edition

The aim of this second edition is still to be an introduction to the restoration of teeth for the undergraduate dental student who is embarking on a practical course in operative dentistry. It is deliberately concise so that it is affordable by students. With the introduction of a longer dental course in the UK, it is disappointing that additional time is not being devoted to clinical dentistry. It is to be hoped that the additional science will make the students better able to think and to question clinical treatment.

Changes have been made in the text to reflect current views and changing ideas, but there have been no radical alterations.

For this edition, I remain grateful to Professor A. H. R. Rowe for his encouragement, advice and provision of facilities. I should also like to thank Dr David Brown and Dr William Saunders for particular advice.

Miss Diane Hogan has carefully wordprocessed the manuscript, Ms Camilla Schierbeck has seen the new edition through the press, and I thank Messrs Peter Saugman and John Harrison of Blackwell Scientific Publications for supporting this book.

My wife and children have been very tolerant while I have spent hours at my desk; for this I am very grateful.

Preface to the first edition

This book is intended to be an introduction to the restoration of teeth for the undergraduate dental student embarking on a practical course of instruction in the subject.

It is no mistake that the book commences with a chapter on dental caries, for the understanding of the disease should be fundamental to treatment, although some texts in the past have covered the disease process in a disproportionately small space. The prevention of dental disease is given prominence because the aim of the dental profession should be to prevent the need for treatment, and furthermore because the success of treatment is short-lived in an environment conducive to disease.

The central section of the book is concerned with conventional treatment of dental caries — that is, cavity preparation and insertion of a restoration. Whilst there has been a decrease in the prevalence of dental caries in the Western World, it is still necessary for students to be competent in operative procedures on qualification, especially with the increasing desire of patients to retain teeth rather than to have them extracted. Considerable emphasis is placed on the use of amalgam, since it has been used by dentists for so many years; whether it will remain the dominent restorative material must be a matter for speculation. The use of composite resins in anterior teeth is described in detail, but at the time of writing the second generation of posterior composites is still in the stage of clinical trials, and in view of previous false starts it would be premature to have included them in the same way in a basic undergraduate text, which must be somewhat conservative.

The latter part covers first the treatment of pulpal disease because it is an integral part of conservative dentistry, but the description is brief because this subject is so well covered in textbooks of endodontics. The final chapter takes the student, who has probably learnt his initial operative dentistry in a laboratory, to the clinical environment, a transition that is often a daunting experience.

The subject of bridgework has deliberately been excluded as the theme of this book is the restoration of individual teeth, and there are several books available that specifically deal with bridges.

Life is one long learning process and the university student must be made to think and to question. Too much of clinical dentistry has been based on empiricism rather than scientific evidence. It is inevitable with the current knowledge explosion that some aspects of this book will become dated and inaccurate within a short period; therefore the student should not believe without question everything which he reads. I am indebted to many research workers and clinicians from whose knowledge and experience I have drawn; some are credited with mention in the bibliographies at the end of each chapter, but the text has deliberately been lightly referenced to make reading easier.

I am very grateful to Professor A. H. R. Rowe for his encouragement advice and provision of facilities; in addition the following colleagues made valuable contributions, Drs D. Brown and Edwina Kidd, Messrs P. Ayling, D. M. Martin and A. A. Robinson, and finally, my wife and my father. I should like to thank a number of people on the Guy's Campus of the United Medical and Dental Schools, Miss T. Lanagan and Miss W. Proctor for many of the line diagrams, Miss J. Hodgkin for the skilled photographic assistance and Miss J. P. Hodgman for the electron micrographs. I am grateful to Dr Edwina Kidd for Figs 1.8 and 1.9, to Messrs S. P. Kariyawasam and K. FitzPatrick for Figs 1.5 and 1.10, and to the Micro-Mega company for permission to reproduce the diagram in Fig. 15.14. In addition, I have been very fortunate in receiving expert technical support, particularly for the chapters on cast and ceramic restorations, from Mr T. Ormiston.

Mrs Irene Grubb has painstakingly typed the manuscript and with good cheer inserted all my alterations.

I am fortunate to have been given the opportunity to write this book by Messrs Robert Campbell and Peter Saugman of Blackwell Scientific Publications, and to have had the sub-editing assistance of Mr James Rivington.

My wife has been very tolerant while I have spent many hours at my desk, and without her understanding and encouragement the task of writing would have foundered.

1 Dental caries — the disease

1.1 Introduction

Dental caries is a widespread disease of civilization and is preventable, yet most people in civilized countries have been affected at some stage in their lives. The prevalence of the disease and the need to treat it have resulted in the creation of a profession that spends the majority of its effort treating the ravages of tooth decay. A knowledge of the aetiology of dental caries and its spread through the tooth provides a scientific basis for prevention and allows a rational approach to the restoration of decayed teeth.

Dental caries, which is of Latin etymology, simply means 'tooth decay' and is characterized by progressive localized destruction of enamel and dentine caused by the metabolic activity of bacterial plaque. The process starts on the surface of the tooth and penetrates into its bulk; when it reaches dentine, it progresses more rapidly and appears to balloon out, undermining enamel.

The way in which decay affects a tooth is essentially very simple, even though the finer details are more complex. There are three necessary components: the tooth, bacterial plaque and a suitable diet. The presence of the first is *sine qua non*, the second is invariably present, but it is the diet which is the main causative factor. A change in diet is the principal reason for an increased incidence of dental caries which has occurred in some communities with the advent of western civilization. The highly cariogenic component of the diet is refined sugar or sucrose, which is metabolized by the bacteria in dental plaque to produce acid which dissolves enamel.

1.2 The carious process

The carious process may be represented diagrammatically as follows:

Substrate + Plaque + Tooth ⟶ Caries
(sugar)   (bacteria) (enamel or   (bacterial   (deminer-
                         dentine)   metabolism)   alization)

It is a sweeping generalization to say that a high sugar intake is the cause of tooth decay, yet it is the most important variable affecting caries activity.

By examining the mechanism of dental caries more closely, an understanding is formed of the contribution of diet, oral hygiene and

1

ways of making the tooth more resistant to decay, together with an appreciation of why certain sites on teeth become affected at different ages.

SUBSTRATE

First, the action of sugars will be considered. Cariogenicity is not the sole prerogative of refined sugars such as sucrose and glucose, but these, and particularly the former, are highly effective. The effect of consuming sugar is to cause a *rapid* drop in plaque pH, which favours enamel demineralization, followed by a *slow* rise in pH. This was first demonstrated by Stephan in 1944, who gave his subjects a rinse of glucose and measured the pH over the following hour, by the end of which the pH had still not returned to the original level. Of great clinical significance is the time for which the pH stays below 5.5, which is regarded as the critical level for demineralization of enamel. The drop in pH for caries-active patients was found to be more than that for caries-free patients and to remain more acidic for longer. Two points emerge: frequency of intake is very significant in caries activity, and caries-prone patients are at greatest risk of further carious attack. Figure 1.1 is a simplified version of Stephan's original diagram.

Sucrose and, to a lesser extent, glucose are metabolized to form both intracellular and extracellular polysaccharides, which allow the bacteria to cling tenaciously to the tooth surface and provide a reservoir of energy for continued cariogenic metabolism as well as proliferation of cariogenic bacteria.

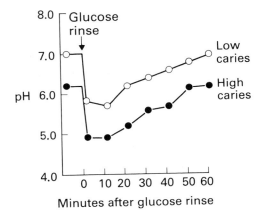

Fig. 1.1 The fall in pH of plaque after a rinse with 10% glucose solution in people with high and low caries activity. Note the rapid fall and slow rise. (After Stephan, 1944.)

PLAQUE

The role of bacteria in causing caries was ascribed to Miller in the 1890s, but proof that their presence is necessary did not come until the 1950s when Orland and his research group in the United States failed to produce caries in germ-free rats fed a cariogenic diet. However, on introducing bacteria to the mouths of these animals, caries ensued. Since their investigation, a number of workers have refined the gnotobiotic techniques, and Fitzgerald, working in collaboration at the US National Institute for Dental Research, has shown that *Streptococcus mutans* is a highly cariogenic micro-organism which produces large amounts of polysaccharide. For many years *Lactobacilli* were considered to be cariogenic; however, most of the gnotobiotic experiments with these bacteria have shown their inability to initiate enamel caries.

Lactobacilli do produce acid and, more importantly, can survive in conditions of low pH and this may explain their frequent observation in carious dentine; they appear to be involved in the destruction of dentine but their role could be more that of passengers than pathogens.

Bacterial plaque is a highly organized structure of bacteria which adheres to the tooth surface. It is usually not difficult to observe plaque on some surfaces of teeth in a patient's mouth. Where plaque is present, the tooth surface appears dull, but plaque may be more readily seen by staining it with a vegetable dye such as erythrocin. Plaque forms on all exposed tooth surfaces and restorations; it proliferates best where it is least disturbed, such as around the gingival margins, on the approximal surfaces and in the fissures. Less is usually found on the cusps because of the combined action of food particles, the tongue and a toothbrush in removing it.

Most patients make some effort to remove plaque but inevitably fail to achieve total success; so it is usual to find certain areas in a patient's mouth with old plaque and other areas with newer plaque. The bacterial content of these plaques differs. In newly formed plaque *Streptococci* and *Neisseria* dominate, but as time progresses other bacteria proliferate, particularly *Actinomyces* and *Veillonella*, so that mature plaque is largely filamentous and contains many more anaerobes.

Almost a third of the plaque is composed of extracellular polysaccharide, which binds the plaque together and sticks it to the tooth surface. It provides a ready store of energy for metabolism to continue long after dietary sugar has been washed away. The plaque acts as a barrier preventing the rapid loss of ions from the tooth and also stopping buffers or ions in the saliva from reaching the tooth surface. The loss of tooth substance in dental caries is a complex process and is markedly different from the effects of acids applied to the tooth surface where mineral is removed from the surface. The carious lesion can be quite advanced before the tooth surface breaks down; the difference appears to be a function of the limitation of ion movement by bacterial plaque.

The elimination of plaque will help to prevent caries and the effect is most marked on the buccal surfaces, which are readily accessible to cleaning. The effect on the approximal surfaces is considerably less pronounced, because toothbrushing alone will not remove all the plaque and only a few patients regularly and effectively use dental floss on these surfaces. The effect on pits and fissures is probably least of all, because toothbrush bristles are usually wider than the fissure and therefore the plaque remains undisturbed.

TOOTH

The last part of the chain to be considered is the tooth surface. It is surprising the number of patients who believe that they are *born* with either strong teeth or soft teeth. Yet the differences between 'soft' and 'strong' teeth are very small or non-existent. It is known that enamel which contains fluoride salts is more resistant to dental caries than enamel which does not. The clinical effect of this in reducing the prevalence of caries is known, but the exact way in which the fluoride ions do this is not clear.

Enamel is composed of crystals of hydroxyapatite arranged in prisms, with traces of fluorapatite particularly near its surface. Any part of the tooth surface can be affected by caries, and this has been demonstrated experimentally. However, clinically, caries usually occurs at specific sites. These may be classified into two major areas: fissures and smooth surfaces.

The fissures in a tooth are usually the first sites to be affected by caries and the disease often commences shortly after eruption. Caries affects the walls of a fissure where it is impossible to remove the plaque with a toothbrush. The beneficial action of fluoride is least in this type of caries.

Caries affecting the smooth surfaces occurs exclusively under bacterial plaque and its incidence is considerably reduced by the action of fluoride.

Caries is normally a slowly progressing disease and its activity is phasic. Until the tooth surface collapses, the demineralization can be partially reversed by the action of saliva, which contains calcium salts and buffers. This remineralization of the tooth is aided by the application of fluoride solutions.

1.3 Occurrence

From the time a tooth erupts, until the time it is lost, all of its exposed surfaces are at risk of caries. However, the pattern of attack is generally predictable.

Caries of fissures occurs soon after tooth eruption and a survey of British children in 1973 showed that within 3 years of eruption the fissures of half of the first permanent molars had been affected (Todd, 1975). The incidence of fissure caries declines as the years after eruption increase, first because the susceptible sites have already succumbed, and secondly because the surface enamel becomes more resistant as fluoride from the diet or toothpaste is continually deposited in the surface layer.

Caries of the approximal surfaces is not usually observed so soon after eruption because it is a sequel to the eruption of adjacent teeth and the surfaces are not then readily visible. By about 6 years after eruption, most of the susceptible approximal surfaces will have succumbed. Therefore, caries is essentially a disease of youth. It is primarily the result of a high sugar diet, which fortunately often improves in adulthood. Children usually have a passion for sweet foods and drinks, and if the frequency of their intake is not controlled, extensive caries can rapidly develop.

Occasionally, people who give up smoking develop a habit of sucking sweets, particularly mints; the result can be a marked rise in caries incidence. Whenever an unexpected rise in the incidence of caries is seen, the cause should be sought.

Older patients are prone to root caries following gingival recession, and the clinician should be particularly observant for these lesions as they may occur in patients who have suffered very little enamel caries.

Because of the large amounts of saliva produced by the submandibular salivary glands, whose ducts open just behind the lower incisors, it is unusual for the lower incisors to be affected by caries.

A small number of patients who suffer from salivary gland insufficiency as a result of disease (Sjögren's syndrome) or are taking certain medicines, e.g. antidepressants, or those who have received radiotherapy are liable to develop an increased incidence of caries shortly after they notice the dry mouth. These patients present a problem to the clinician. Particular attention must be paid to careful dietary control and scrupulous oral hygiene. It is most helpful if there is close liaison between the dentist and doctor from the outset of medical treatment in order to prevent the development of carious lesions. The patient who has received radiotherapy may, not unnaturally, have been preoccupied with the tumour which needed treatment and so have neglected his teeth. However, tooth loss should be avoided because of the risk of osteomyelitis in irradiated bone, and because dentures are not well tolerated in dry mouths; therefore, the patient must be encouraged to resume an interest in his teeth.

Unless the early lesion in enamel is arrested, caries is usually a progressive disease, but the rate of progress is very variable. Particularly in children, lesions can progress from being undetectable to needing treatment within a year; in adults, lesions may remain virtually static for a number of years; but in both, the reverse is quite possible.

Once caries has commenced, the tooth is damaged for ever, yet if the early lesion is arrested soon enough, it is far preferable to leave a chalky enamel surface alone than to treat the caries by placing a restoration. There are many adults whose teeth show evidence of early carious lesions which commenced in their youth but have not progressed, because their diet is now favourable and oral hygiene measures are effective.

A measure of the patient's susceptibility to caries may be established by counting the number of teeth which are decayed, missing or filled. This is known as the DMF index. It is a crude index because it takes no account of the number of surfaces affected by caries, it can be inflated by tooth loss through other causes, especially in older patients, and it may be influenced by treatment patterns. A better index is the DMFS, which takes into account the number of surfaces affected by disease or restored. Even with the DMFS there is no distinction between the earliest sign of caries and severe caries. Therefore, in a number of research investigations, particularly into the effect of fluoride toothpastes, only caries affecting approximal surfaces has been measured using solely radiographic examination. Where the *prevalence* of caries has been measured at two different times in the same individual, the *incidence* of new lesions can be found.

It is by the use of indices in epidemiological studies that evidence has accumulated of the declining prevalence of caries in many countries during the 1970s, recently shown in the Children's Dental Health Survey of 1983 in the United Kingdom (OPCS, 1983).

SITES OF CARIES

There are four main sites of carious attack:
1   A fissured enamel surface.
2   A smooth enamel surface.
3   The root surface.
4   Adjacent to a restoration.

Fissure caries

The attack of fissures by caries is the most common form of the disease and the fissure is usually the first site of caries on a tooth. Fissures frequently become carious within a few years of eruption and if they do not become carious in the high risk period, the chances of their developing caries thereafter are low.

The fissure forms a good nidus for plaque and it is extremely difficult to remove plaque from a fissure as toothbrush bristles cannot get into any but the widest. Caries starts on both walls of a fissure — not at its base as was previously thought — and spreads into the enamel. On reaching the amelo-dentinal junction it spreads more rapidly along the junction and into dentine. The clinician is frequently

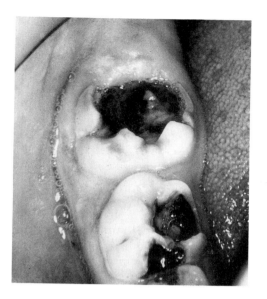

Fig. 1.2 Extensive occlusal caries causing destruction of the clinical crown of a lower first molar. The deciduous molar in front has large mesial and occlusal carious lesions.

confronted with a fissure that superficially appears to be only slightly carious, but when it is examined radiographically and access is gained to the carious dentine, he is surprised by the extent of the disease. It is relatively late in the disease process that the enamel collapses to form a clinically observable cavity. If fissure caries is treated, usually by cavity preparation and insertion of a restoration, before extensive dentine involvement occurs, the cavity can be kept small and the remaining tooth is not weakened. Extensive occlusal caries results in a weakened tooth, with cusps and enamel walls liable to fracture. Untreated fissure caries may lead to destruction of the clinical crown of the tooth (Fig. 1.2).

Smooth surface

This type of caries occurs on surfaces where there has been an extensive build-up of plaque for some time.

A very common site is the approximal surface cervical to the contact, and caries may occur following the eruption of adjacent teeth. The size of the enamel lesion is determined by the extent of the plaque and clinical breakdown of enamel may be observed relatively sooner compared with fissure caries. However, its detection on the approximal surface in a clinical examination is often hampered by the presence of the adjacent tooth. On reaching dentine, the lesion spreads along the amelo-dentinal junction as well as into the dentine. In time, the enamel marginal ridge becomes unsupported by sound dentine, and collapses. By this stage the lesion will be large and the pulp endangered; it is beyond the optimum size for treatment. This type of lesion on posterior teeth is best detected using radiography.

Smooth surface caries may occur at another site of plaque accumulation, the gingival border of enamel. It is readily detected by removing the plaque, and noting chalky enamel or loss of surface contour. It is a sign of poor oral hygiene and a diet with a high sugar intake. Where the disease is localized to the buccal surfaces of the lower teeth, it often indicates a habit of sucking sweets or mints. Treatment must consist not only of removing the caries but also of correcting the diet and oral hygiene procedures; the former without the latter will always be unsuccessful.

Root caries

This type of caries affects older patients whose gingivae have receded and may arise on the roots of teeth whose enamel has not succumbed to caries. Because there is no surface enamel, caries involving the

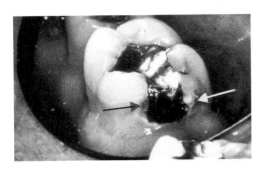

Fig. 1.3 Recurrent caries in the enamel on the approximal surface buccal and lingual to an amalgam restoration in a lower molar.

cementum and dentine can become established within a short period. The pulp is closer to the surface of the root than it is in the crown, so pulpal involvement may arise while the lesion still appears small. Where these lesions occur on the approximal surface, the clinician may fail to notice them until they are larger than the optimum size for treatment. Such a cavity may be associated with a poor approximal contact which has allowed food packing, and where the patient has periodontal pocketing the cavity may be obscured by the soft tissues.

Caries around restorations

It would be incorrect to assume that once a restoration has been placed in a tooth, caries could not recur on the restored surfaces. Recurrent caries around metallic restorations is the most common cause of their replacement (Fig. 1.3).

Further spread of caries may be seen because the original lesion was inadequately treated, the restoration did not completely fill the cavity allowing a nidus for plaque accumulation, or inadequate plaque and dietary control continued after the restoration had been placed. A new lesion may occur on the tooth surface adjacent to the restoration or on the wall of the cavity against the restoration.

It is therefore necessary to examine the margins of restorations in a patient's mouth to observe if caries is occurring at these sites.

CLASSIFICATION

The sites at which caries occurs were classified by Dr G. V. Black at the turn of the century. His classification was based on the order of attack of the surfaces of the teeth, and is still widely used in dental schools even though it does not identify the affected surfaces.

Class

1 Caries affecting pits and fissures.
2 Caries affecting the approximal surfaces of posterior teeth.
3 Caries affecting the approximal surfaces of anterior teeth.
4 Caries affecting the approximal surfaces of anterior teeth and involving the incisal angle.
5 Caries affecting the cervical surfaces.

Black's classification of lesions is frequently applied, incorrectly, to the restorations that are required to treat these lesions.

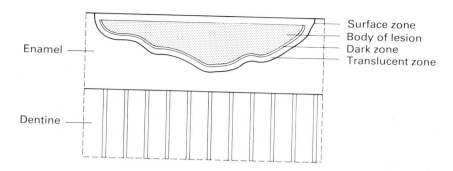

Fig. 1.4 Diagram of a smooth surface carious lesion in enamel showing the four zones.

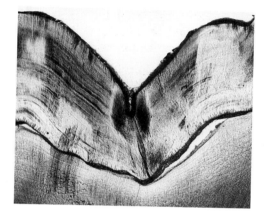

Fig. 1.5 Longitudinal ground section of a tooth showing carious lesions in enamel on either side of a fissure.

1.4 Pathology of enamel caries

Treatment can only be applied rationally when the disease is understood, therefore enamel caries will be covered in detail. All lesions, wherever they arise on enamel, can be reduced to a single type, the smooth surface lesion (Fig. 1.4), because fissure caries is simply two smooth surface lesions on opposite walls of the fissure (Fig. 1.5). Recurrent caries is still a smooth surface lesion which may be on the outer surface of the tooth or on the enamel wall against the restoration (Fig. 1.6).

The earliest sign of caries may be seen as a white spot when the plaque has been removed. The size of the white spot is related to the extent of the cariogenic plaque, and may cover a large area. It is distinguishable from the surrounding enamel by its greater opacity (Fig. 1.7). The surface of the tooth is entirely smooth and indeed the perikymata may be readily observed. If the tooth was sectioned and a ground section examined in polarized light, the lesion could be divided into four zones (Figs 1.4, 1.8 & 1.9): the translucent zone, the dark zone, the body of the lesion and the surface zone.

Fig. 1.6 Diagram of recurrent caries which may occur on the tooth surface adjacent to the restoration or on the cavity wall.

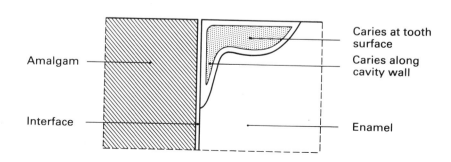

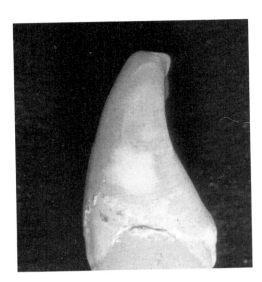

Fig. 1.7 The earliest sign of caries is seen as a white opaque spot on the enamel; the enamel surface appears intact.

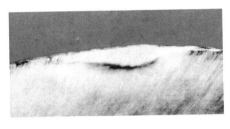

Fig. 1.8 Longitudinal ground section of an enamel lesion examined in quinoline. A translucent zone may be seen at the advancing front of the lesion, superficial to which is the dark zone. The body of the lesion appears translucent.

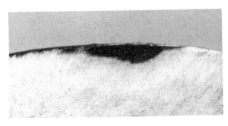

Fig. 1.9 The same section as Fig. 1.8 examined in water with polarized light showing the thin surface zone over the body of the lesion.

TRANSLUCENT ZONE

This is the advancing front of the lesion and indicates a 1% loss of mineral. It is frequently observed when the section is immersed in quinoline.

DARK ZONE

This is a thin band superficial to the translucent zone and appears dark in quinoline because the quinoline cannot enter some of the smaller pores created by demineralization. Mineral loss is 2–4%.

BODY OF LESION

This accounts for the bulk of the lesion and is translucent in quinoline. Mineral loss is up to 25% and may also be observed on microradiographs (radiographs of ground sections).

SURFACE ZONE

This is the relatively intact surface layer of enamel which is radiopaque on a microradiograph. This zone is not detectable when the section is in quinoline but may be seen when it is immersed in water. Mineral loss is less than 4%. The zone is approximately 30 μm wide and occurs even on surfaces where the original tooth surface had been removed prior to initiation of caries.

The early enamel lesion is characterized by the surface layer remaining intact and demineralization occurring within the enamel. Enamel caries is a slowly progressing phasic process which is partially reversible. If a mineralizing solution is applied to the surface of the lesion, the deeper layers will remineralize.

The lesion so far described has an intact surface and so microorganisms have penetrated into the tooth. The lesion is cone-shaped with its base at the enamel surface and the apex deep in the enamel. The late enamel lesion still with an intact surface may be arrested by suitable dietary and plaque control. Some remineralization will occur given favourable conditions; therefore, such a lesion should not be treated by cavity preparation.

When the lesion reaches the amelo-dentinal junction, a dentinal response occurs before cavitation of the enamel surface.

1.5 Pathology of dentine caries

On reaching the dentine, demineralization spreads along the amelo-dentinal junction and then into the dentine on a broad front. Spread

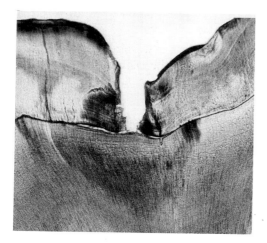

Fig. 1.10 Longitudinal ground section of a tooth showing caries with loss of enamel exposing dentine. The amelo-dentinal junction is involved for some distance either side of the fissure. The deep spread of the lesion into dentine is affected by the orientation of dentinal tubules.

into the dentine is affected by the orientation of the dentinal tubules (Fig. 1.10).

EARLY DENTINE LESION

When caries first affects dentine the enamel surface is usually still intact. The surface dentine becomes demineralized and the odontoblasts, the processes of which extend about a third of the way into the dentinal tubules from the pulp, react to the lowered pH at the tubule extremities with two main responses, tubular sclerosis and formation of reactionary dentine.

Tubular sclerosis is an accelerated form of peritubular dentine formation, but the process continues further than normal as the tubules become completely blocked with apatite crystals. This sclerosis protects the underlying odontoblasts from the advancing caries, and occurs at the distal extremities of the odontoblast processes. If sclerotic dentine is examined in a ground section by transmitted light, it appears transparent compared with the remainder of the dentine where the light is scattered by the tubules. In a radiograph of a ground section, it appears more radiopaque than the rest of the dentine.

Reactionary dentine is an accelerated form of regular secondary dentine which, because of its faster formation, is less regular, and it is only formed by the odontoblast layer under the tubules affected by caries (Fig 1.11).

LATER DENTINE LESION

If the carious lesion progresses further, the enamel surface will collapse, allowing bacteria to enter the enamel, and the rate of decay

Fig. 1.11 Diagram of an advanced carious lesion in dentine showing the zones of destruction, penetration and demineralization as well as the tubular sclerosis and reactionary dentine formed.

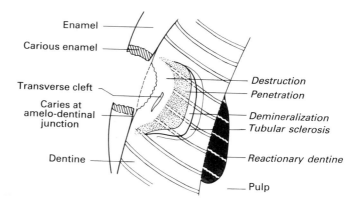

increases. The bacteria soon invade the dentine and grow down the tubules.

The dentine lesion may then be divided into three zones (Fig. 1.11): the zone of demineralization, the zone of penetration and the zone of destruction.

Demineralized zone

This is the advancing front of the lesion in which there are no bacteria. Most likely none are found because the conditions are too acidic for the micro-organisms to survive, and the supply of nutrients is poor because the pulpal ends of the tubules are sealed by sclerotic dentine.

Zone of penetration

Bacteria are found in this zone growing in chains along the tubules. *Lactobacilli* predominate and this is probably as much a reflection of their ability to survive in acidic conditions as their ability to produce acid. *Lactobacilli* are found in low numbers in plaque on the tooth surface and have been shown not to cause enamel caries, but they may be involved in the destruction of dentine.

Zone of destruction

The structure of the dentine is destroyed by proteolytic enzymes from the mixed bacterial flora breaking down the collagen matrix. Bacterial invasion is extensive, particularly in the shrinkage clefts within the affected dentine. This dentine is very soft and can be readily removed from the cavity by hand excavators.

The dentine lesion can be excavated away to reveal the hard sclerotic dentine which formed a barrier.

EXTENSIVE DENTINE LESION

As the dentine lesion continues to progress, sound enamel at the periphery of the carious enamel ceases to be supported by sound dentine and may collapse, particularly if it is subjected to occlusal forces, revealing the far more extensive dentine lesion.

The zone of demineralization advances further through the primary sclerotic dentine to affect the underlying odontoblasts, which endeavour to retreat by laying down more reactionary dentine; this layer of dentine is likely to be very irregular in the attempt to seal off the tubules and protect the odontoblasts. The success of this defence will depend on it being more rapid than the progress of the carious lesion. As the lesion expands, odontoblasts decrease in number so few are found under the reactionary dentine.

The next change is inflammation of the pulp, and is seen when bacteria are found in the tubules within 1 mm of the pulp. There is a characteristic infiltrate of chronic inflammatory cells in the pulp under the affected tubules. The odontoblast layer does not survive long with bacteria so close in the dentine, and once cellular necrosis occurs, inflammation is likely to be irreversible. When the bacteria almost reach the pulp, acute inflammation supervenes and its extent is likely to be limited to the affected pulp horn. Polymorphonuclear leucocytes will be observed in the pulp horn, with loss of normal tissue structure. This is followed by formation of a micro-abscess. When carious dentine is excavated, softened dentine can be scraped away to expose a small aperture into the pulp chamber, a carious exposure; from it, frequently emerges a bead of pus. The tooth may not necessarily have caused the patient pain by this stage.

Infection of the pulp is a late event in the carious process and can eventually spread through the radicular pulp to cause infection in the periapical bone, a periapical abscess. This is accompanied by severe pain, tenderness of the affected tooth, swelling of the alveolus and face and, on occasion, general malaise. A periapical abscess is now not such a common sequel to caries because tooth decay is often treated before involvement of the pulp.

An alternative reaction to abscess formation in the pulp is necrosis, which is initially limited to that part under the carious dentine but may eventually spread to involve the entire pulp; it is symptomless unless infection supervenes.

1.6 Diagnosis of caries

CLINICAL METHODS

Clinical methods of diagnosis are: direct visual examination, transillumination, use of a dental probe and use of dental floss.

Direct visual examination

The tooth must be *dried* and any covering of plaque removed before it can be examined properly.

The earliest sign of caries is a white spot on the enamel. The enamel still has a normal contour, although this is not normally observable on the approximal surface because the adjacent tooth ob-

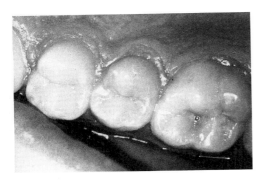

Fig. 1.12 A small carious lesion in the central fossa of an upper molar showing discoloration of the dentine through the enamel around the fossa. Cavity preparation is required.

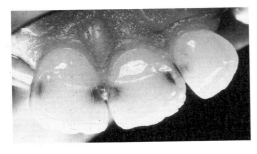

Fig. 1.13 Approximal carious lesions in upper anterior teeth seen by transillumination as dark shadows extending into dentine.

structs access. In the depth of a carious fissure the enamel walls may appear chalky white.

A later sign of caries is loss of surface contour. This is readily observable on the buccal and lingual surfaces, less so on the occlusal surface, and rarely on the approximal surface because of the presence of the adjacent tooth.

With dentine involvement, carious dentine will appear a different colour from normal dentine which is off-white/ivory. The carious dentine usually appears yellow/brown although in the older and more slowly progressing lesion it can appear blue/black. Carious dentine may be seen directly where there is no enamel, or indirectly through sound enamel around affected fissures (Fig. 1.12), and also through approximal marginal ridges where the spreading lesion in dentine from the approximal surface is close to the marginal ridge.

With continued progress of the dentine lesion the underside of the enamel may become demineralized and this can give an opaque white appearance to the enamel.

Collapse of enamel through lack of support is a late event and indicates extensive caries of dentine. This amount of caries is readily detectable, and by this stage there may possibly be pulpal involvement (Fig. 1.2).

Transillumination

If light is allowed to pass through the tooth, a carious lesion will appear as a dark shadow. This is widely used to detect approximal lesions in anterior teeth (Fig. 1.13). It is a less useful method for posterior teeth because the teeth are broader and because the operating light, which is the usual source of light, is not suitably positioned. With the increasing availability of intraoral fibre-optic lights, transillumination of posterior teeth may become more widespread.

Use of a dental probe

The probe may be used to follow the contour of the tooth surface and to detect softening due to caries in pits and fissures. Where the surface enamel on the walls of a fissure has cavitated, the probe will, under light pressure, wedge into the softened enamel. Care should be taken to differentiate cavitation caused by caries from a fissure that is anatomically deep but non-carious; in the former the enamel in the fissure will appear chalky white with a surrounding dentine shadow, while in the latter the tooth will be of normal appearance. With carious destruction of dentine under a fissure and loss of overlying enamel, a probe will readily penetrate into dentine, stick and require some effort to be withdrawn. On the approximal surface a small hooked probe (Briault) is particularly useful as access to a standard probe is restricted.

A probe is also used to detect deficiencies and caries around existing restorations by observing whether it penetrates the junction and, if so, how far. In the absence of visible demineralization, penetration up to 0.5 mm without sticking does not normally indicate the need for treatment. However, if it penetrates more and becomes stuck between the restoration and the surrounding tooth, caries is usually present.

The probe must not be used as a substitute for careful visual examination of a tooth which has been dried. When used with heavy pressure, it may even destroy the intact surface zone of a white spot lesion which could otherwise have been remineralized. For this reason, some clinicians deprecate the use of a probe.

Use of dental floss

This may be run over the approximal surface and, if it frays, it is indicative of ragged enamel margins of a carious cavity, the rough edge of an existing restoration, or calculus.

RADIOGRAPHY

X-rays are absorbed by mineralized tissue and therefore when a source of X-rays is directed at the teeth an image will be produced on a film placed behind them. Loss of mineral caused by caries will affect the image produced on the film, and use of this is made to detect carious lesions, particularly on the approximal surfaces.

The type of radiograph which best demonstrates approximal caries is a bitewing film (Fig. 1.14). The X-ray beam passes horizontally through the crowns of the teeth at right angles to the line of the teeth being examined. Detection of caries is more difficult if the beam passes obliquely, as may occur when the beam is carelessly aligned or a periapical view is used. The radiographic image is a two-dimensional shadow produced by a three-dimensional structure, the tooth. The image on the developed radiograph is dependent on a number of variables, i.e. the source of radiation, the film, the process of developing of the film, and the amount and type of tissue through which the X-rays pass. Therefore, radiographs should be interpreted with caution and the operator must be aware that clinically detectable lesions may not necessarily be observable on radiographs. The radiographic examination should therefore *follow* and not precede or replace the clinical examination.

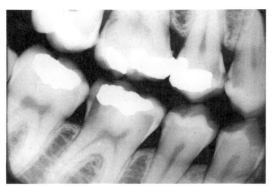 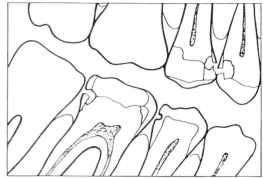

Fig. 1.14 *Left*: bitewing radiograph of right posterior teeth. *Right*: diagram of radiograph. An enamel lesion is seen on distal surface of tooth 45. Extensive dentine lesions are seen on 46 (distal), 14 (distal) and 15 (mesial) with accompanying enamel lesions. There is a dentine lesion on 46 (mesial) without an enamel lesion being obvious. FDI tooth rotation has been used (p. 234).

The detection on a radiograph of all but the largest lesions on the buccal and lingual surfaces of a tooth is difficult because of the relatively small loss of mineral compared with the bulk of the tooth. Similarly, enamel caries in a fissure is not observable, but once dentine involvement becomes extensive it is possible to observe an area of radiolucency in the dentine at the base of the fissure. Occlusal caries may be detected radiographically when it has not been observed clinically; this is more likely to occur in teeth which have naturally opaque enamel and in teeth where topical application of fluoride has remineralized enamel stopping it from collapsing although there is bacterial penetration of dentine. Sawle and Andlaw (1988) have reported that since the use of fluoride toothpaste became widespread, occlusal caries has become harder to detect clinically.

The approximal lesion is most readily detected on a good quality bitewing radiograph, and is often observed before there is clinical evidence of a lesion because the surface is obstructed from visual examination by the adjacent tooth. There are two components to the radiographic lesion: the enamel radiolucency and the dentine radiolucency (Fig. 1.14). The enamel radiolucency indicates a carious lesion in enamel and is visible before the surface of the tooth cavitates. The size of the enamel radiolucency may change little while the dentine radiolucency expands considerably. Rugg-Gunn (1972) showed that when there was a radiolucency in the enamel up to the amelo-dentinal junction but not one in dentine, half of the enamel surfaces which he examined were still intact. Therefore, the clinician should not automatically consider that the tooth must be restored when an enamel lesion is seen on a radiograph. It is possible to prevent the lesion from progressing by a suitable preventive regime. The radiograph does not disclose whether the lesion is active or quiescent; and it would be necessary to look back over previous radiographs to see whether the lesion had remained static or increased in size.

The dentine radiolucency denotes caries of dentine and normally indicates the need for cavity preparation and restoration, because such a lesion usually progresses and non-intervention may lead to avoidable pulpal disease. The dentine radiolucency is a darker shade of grey on a radiograph than sound dentine, is not readily visible and tends to merge into the sound dentine towards the body of the tooth, and often the carious lesion is larger than the radiograph suggests. The radiographic lesion is approximately semicircular with its flat surface against the enamel. The dentine radiolucency is seen best when it is in conjunction with an enamel radiolucency that has penetrated through to dentine. However, in a number of teeth it is not possible to observe an enamel radiolucency because the X-ray beam has been obstructed by so much sound enamel either side of the lesion; yet there is a very definite radiolucency in dentine and furthermore the carious lesion is in need of treatment. Rugg-Gunn (1972) showed that half of the teeth that displayed advanced white spot lesions in enamel when examined appeared normal on radiographs.

Care must be taken not to confuse the natural radiolucency at the neck of the tooth with caries. The neck of the tooth approximally appears darker because there is little or no overlying enamel, the tooth is narrower and there is no overlying alveolar bone. In many young patients the neck of the tooth is not exposed to plaque but covered by sulcular epithelium or periodontal fibres, depending on the position.

On a radiograph it is possible for the shadow of the carious lesion in dentine to be superimposed over that of the pulp chamber; it does not automatically indicate that caries has spread to the pulp.

Bibliography

Black G. V. (1917) *A Work on Operative Dentistry*, 3rd edn, Vol. 1. Medico-Dental Publishing Co., Chicago.

Fitzgerald R. J. & Keyes R. H. (1960) Demonstration of the aetiologic role of Streptococci in experimental caries in the hamster. *Journal of the American Dental Association*, **61**, 9–19.

Grey P. G., Todd J. E., Slack G. L. & Bulman J. S. (1970) *Adult Dental Health in England and Wales 1968*. HMSO, London.

Miller (1890) *The Microorganisms of the Human Mouth.* S.S. White, Philadelphia.

OPCS (1983) *Children's Dental Health 1983.* OPCS Monitor SS 83/2. HMSO, London. (Reprinted in *British Dental Journal*, **155**, 322–328.)

Orland F. J., Blayney J. R., Harrison R. W., Reyniers J. A. Trexler P. C., Gordon H. A., Wagner M. & Lockey T. D. (1954) Use of germ-free animal technique in the study of experimental dental caries. *Journal of Dental Research*, **33**, 147–174.

Rugg-Gunn A. J. (1972) Approximal carious lesions. *British Dental Journal*, **133**, 481–484.

Sawle R. F. & Andlaw R. J. (1988) Has occlusal caries become more difficult to diagnose? *British Dental Journal*, **164**, 209–211.

Silverstone L. M. (1968) The surface zone in caries and in caries-like lesions produced *in vitro. British Dental Journal*, **125**, 145–157.

Silverstone L. M., Johnson N. W., Hardie J. M. & Williams R. A. D. (1981) *Dental Caries, Aetiology, Pathology and Prevention*, Part I, pp. 1–206. Macmillan, London.

Smith N. J. D. (1988) *Dental Radiography*, 2nd edn. Blackwell Scientific Publications, Oxford.

Stephan R. M. (1944) Intraoral hydrogen ion concentrations — associated with dental caries activity. *Journal of Dental Research*, **23**, 254–266.

Todd J. E. (1975) *Children's Dental Health in England and Wales 1973.* HMSO London.

2 Prevention and control of dental caries

2.1 Introduction

The principal aim of the dentist should be to prevent dental disease, and having examined the pathology of dental caries in the previous chapter, a rational basis for preventing it can now be formulated.

Prevention can be divided into three stages. First, there is primary prevention of the disease, i.e. not developing dental caries at all. Secondly, there is the control of early lesions and preventing their enlargement to the size where restorations become necessary. Thirdly, there is the prevention of recurrent caries around existing restorations so that they do not fail prematurely.

Many dentists in the past did not devote sufficient time to preventing dental caries, mainly because there was so much disease to treat; however, the prevention and control of this disease is fundamental to the long-term survival of teeth and restorations placed in them. Before a restoration is placed in a tooth, the disease must be controlled or the life of the restoration will be very limited.

Preventive measures may be applied to each of the three components — substrate, plaque and tooth — may be of a general or specific nature. In brief they can be summarized as shown in Table 2.1. General preventive measures are performed outside the dental surgery and do not actively involve the dentist, while the specific measures involve the dentist or his assistants.

Table 2.1 Summary of prevention of dental caries.

	Substrate	Plaque	Tooth
General preventive measures	Dietary advice Sugar substitutes	Oral hygiene Mouthwashes Vaccination	Systemic fluoride Fluoride toothpastes Fluoride mouthrinses
Specific control measures	Dietary counselling	Plaque control programme	Fluoride application Tissue sealants Restorations

2.2 General preventive measures

SUBSTRATE REGULATION

The harmful effects of regular intake of sugar, particularly sucrose, have already been mentioned and this was shown in detail in the

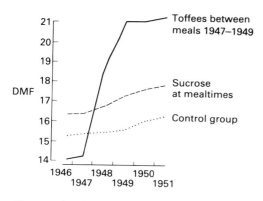

Fig. 2.1 The effects of sugar consumption on the number of decayed, missing or filled teeth from the Vipeholm study. Sugar in the form of toffees consumed between meals caused a marked increase in caries. (After Gustafsson *et al.*, 1954.)

Vipeholm study carried out in Sweden during the late 1940s. When sugar was consumed between meals the frequency of new carious lesions was far higher than when it was restricted to mealtimes (Fig. 2.1); further, the sugar content of what was eaten at mealtimes made little difference to the incidence of caries. If this message can be conveyed to patients and especially mothers of young children, then a substantial amount of caries can be prevented solely by control of diet. If children are brought up without sweetened food and drinks either between meals or as a nightcap, then the pattern for later life is established; however, once they have been introduced to such sweetened food then they are naturally reluctant to give it up. The saying 'What they have not had, they will not miss' contains a great deal of truth.

The substitution of fresh fruit or plain crisps for sweets and biscuits consumed as snacks between meals is a positive first step to the elimination of all snacks between meals. Dried fruit should be avoided as a snack because of its high sugar content. Highly processed starchy snacks have also been shown to be cariogenic, as have the flavourings on some crisps. Fruit drinks without added sugar do contain natural sugar. Frequent consumption will lead to caries, therefore the only effective way to prevent caries is to avoid snacks and fruit drinks between meals.

An alternative approach, where the patient continues to consume the wrong things at the wrong times, is the substitution of a less cariogenic sweetener for sucrose. Whilst this is fine for dentists to demand, the processed food industry needs to pass on the increased cost of the alternative sweetener to the public, who prefer the conventional and cheaper natural product. The food industry also takes far more note of the sugar producers who have a very forceful lobby and, to a lesser extent, the medical profession which is not principally interested in dental health. Despite this opposition from the sugar producers, some progress has been made. Saccharin is a non-cariogenic intense sweetener but it does not taste as pleasant as sugar, and patients use it more often because of concern about their weight rather than dental caries. Some 'diet' foods contain saccharin but not all are sugar-free; therefore, changing to these may not be the solution for patients with high rates of caries. A newer sweetener, which patients may buy and which is now included in low-calorie drinks, is aspartame and it has a less bitter taste than saccharin. However, one commercial aspartame sweetener is not sugar-free because it was marketed for slimmers. Xylitol is a bulk sweetener substitute for sugar that has been used in processed foods for diabetics and has been tested extensively in Finland; it is palatable and non-cariogenic, but the main drawbacks to its widescale use are its higher cost and unavailability to the general public.

PLAQUE CONTROL

The removal of plaque will help to prevent caries, but many patients are ignorant of its presence on their teeth. It may be readily seen when it is stained with a disclosing solution. A number of such solutions or soluble tablets are commercially available from retail chemists for patients to use at home.

The extent of plaque on the visible tooth surfaces can be measured using a plaque index; that of Greene & Vermillion is widely used:

0   None present.
1   Plaque covers <1/3 of the tooth.
2   Plaque covers <2/3 of the tooth.
3   Plaque covers >2/3 of the tooth.

The greater the extent of plaque, the greater is the potential threat of caries and gingivitis.

The removal of plaque by mechanical devices, such as a toothbrush, dental floss or a toothpick, can at best only remove plaque from accessible sites. The buccal and lingual surfaces can most easily be kept completely free from plaque, and so effective oral hygiene measures alone can prevent any carious lesions occurring on these surfaces. However, the reduction in caries on other surfaces attributable to oral hygiene procedures must be questionable, particularly as very few patients carry out the procedures efficiently. Indeed, the more enthusiastic patient can do more harm than good by being careless. Dental floss ill used may strip the epithelial attachment, causing damage to the gingivae. Vigorous brushing towards the gingival margin can lead to recession, as can horizontal brushing which, accompanied by an abrasive toothpaste, may also result in wear of the tooth at its neck forming an abrasion cavity. Brushing teeth with water is unexciting for the patient and therefore is likely to be brief. However, the use of a suitably flavoured toothpaste makes the procedure pleasant, so prolonging cleaning and therefore the effectiveness. Most toothpastes are now of low abrasivity to minimize damage to the tooth surface.

The major advertising campaigns on television by toothpaste manufacturers must have made the general public considerably more tooth conscious and have encouraged oral hygiene. Perhaps the greatest benefit of good oral hygiene is the prevention of periodontal disease, and its value lies in being done well rather than often.

Plaque may also be controlled by chemical means, such as antiseptics and in particular chlorhexidine (ICI Pharmaceuticals, Macclesfield, Cheshire). Chlorhexidine as a twice daily mouthwash has been shown to be effective in reducing the growth of plaque on teeth in a number of studies. It has a broad spectrum of antibacterial activity and *Streptococcus mutans* is particularly susceptible to it. Chlorhexidine appears to bind to salivary protein and so approximately 30% of a mouthrinse is retained in the mouth, and this considerably prolongs the time for which it is effective. Plaque is controlled for only as many days as the mouthwash method is used, and following its discontinuation, plaque reforms. The use of a chlorhexidine mouthwash regime is unlikely to be adopted as a long-term anti-caries measure because it has drawbacks. The mouthwash has an unpleasant rather bitter taste and, with continued use, an unsightly brown stain may form on the surfaces of teeth, especially where tooth-brushing is inefficient. The long-term use of an antiseptic has been questioned in relation to the overgrowth of other micro-organisms; however, this appears to be more a theoretical than a real problem.

As dental caries is principally, if not exclusively, caused by *Streptococcus mutans*, it is possible to immunize the individual against the micro-organism. This has been done in experimental animals with some success and in time could be applied to man. A problem with all vaccination procedures is occasional morbidity; this has resulted in many mothers refusing vaccination of their children against serious illnesses such as whooping cough. Dental caries rarely causes serious illness so there may be significant resistance by parents even if the vaccine is proved successful in man.

ALTERED TOOTH

Water fluoridation

The presence of fluoride ions in surface enamel makes it more resistant to dental caries. It has been clearly shown that children brought up in areas with a fluoride level close to or above 1 ppm in the water supply have a lower incidence of caries than those in areas with lower levels of fluoride. When fluoride levels in the water are in excess of 1 ppm there is little further reduction in caries and the teeth are more likely to be formed with blemished, mottled enamel. Therefore, some areas with higher concentrations of fluoride ions in their water supplies have had the levels reduced to approximately 1 ppm. Also, in many parts of the world fluoride has been added to raise the level to 1 ppm. In Britain during the early 1940s, Weaver demonstrated that the caries experience in South Shields (water fluoride level 1.4 ppm) was half that in North Shields (water fluoride level 0.25 ppm). Despite the obvious benefit of adjusting the fluoride level to optimum in all water supplies, only 10% of the population in Britain is so fortunate. This has arisen because the decision to fluoridate is made by local authorities who have not given the issue priority, and secondly because a vociferous minority who regard it as an intrusion of civil liberty have effectively opposed water fluoridation.

Water fluoridation substantially increases the resistance of teeth to caries when they are forming and the enhanced protection is lifelong. The effect of water fluoridation on teeth which have already erupted is less but still beneficial. The measure is principally of benefit to the young but is also of value to adults because of its topical effect in encouraging remineralization of carious enamel.

Birmingham was fluoridated in the mid-1960s and the dental health of its children has now improved so much that students at the dental school need to travel to see caries in deciduous teeth!

Fluoride toothpaste

The use of toothpastes containing fluoride is a way of incorporating fluoride ions into teeth where the fluoride level of the water supply is low. The scale of fluoride toothpaste manufacture is such that it is now difficult to buy fluoride-free toothpaste in Britain. A large number of studies have been conducted into the effectiveness of different fluoride salts in toothpastes. The reduction in caries has been reported as being about 30% and the various trials have been reviewed by Murray & Rugg-Gunn (1982).

However, since it became difficult to buy any other toothpaste, most young children are now using a fluoride toothpaste and this is starting before they are 2 years old. Because of its attractive flavour children use it regularly, and toddlers who cannot spit ingest far more than was ever envisaged and therefore fluoride becomes incorporated into forming teeth. This could be an important factor in the recent reduction of dental caries.

The Children's Dental Health Survey of 1983 in the United Kingdom (OPCS, 1983) has shown a reduction in the number of decayed teeth in children of a comparable age with those in the previous survey of 1973. The regular application of fluoride toothpaste, which provides little fluoride often, to enamel surfaces undergoing the initial stages of demineralization may contribute significantly to remineralization and therefore to the arrest of such lesions.

Fluoride tablets, drops and mouthrinses

Where the water supply is not fluoridated, children may be given fluoride daily either as tablets or drops; dosages are detailed in Table 2.2 — these are lower than previously suggested in order to prevent excessive intake, which in the recent past has led to an increased incidence of mottled enamel. It should be noted that 2.2 mg sodium fluoride contains 1 mg fluoride. To be effective, the fluoride supplement must be given continuously for a number of years and whilst many parents start full of enthusiasm only a few persevere.

Table 2.2 Daily dosage of fluoride supplement in milligrams (from Dowell & Joyston-Bechal, 1981).

Age (years)	Existing fluoride level in water (ppm)		
	<0.3	0.3–0.7	>0.7
<2	0.25	0	0
2–4	0.50	0.25	0
5–16	1.00	0.50	0

Fluoride mouthrinses may be prescribed to patients who are at particular risk of caries. These may be patients with a caries problem or those who have a dry mouth as a result of salivary gland disease or radiotherapy.

2.3 Specific control measures

These measures are carried out in the dental surgery and are usually provided on an individual basis as part of dental care, and increasingly instead of conventional treatment. Whilst they can be given by the dentist, they are often provided by dental hygienists and dental therapists.

DIETARY COUNSELLING

Where the patient's teeth have recently been affected by caries, the diet should be investigated for cariogenic components and particularly frequency of intake *prior* to undertaking the restoration of carious teeth. Such information can be recorded on a diet sheet on which the patient writes down everything that he eats and drinks at, and particularly between, meals for a period of several days. The diet sheet can then be discussed with the patient at the next visit and advice given on how the diet should be adjusted. The use of the diet sheet should be resumed after several weeks to ensure that the advice is being followed. Until it is, the environment is unsuitable for the placement of restorations. Dietary counselling is often carried out in conjunction with instruction in oral hygiene. It is important to counsel in a constructive manner and not to appear to criticize.

PLAQUE CONTROL

The presence of plaque should be demonstrated to the patient by using a disclosing solution, and he should be advised how to remove it using a suitable brush or dental floss as is appropriate for the site, mouth and patient. The plaque levels must be reassessed at the following visit and the patient must be praised for areas where there has been improvement; he must also be encouraged to try harder in areas where there has been inadequate improvement. Particular emphasis should be placed on plaque associated with dental caries, although plaque associated with gingivitis should not be overlooked.

These specific measures are important for the long-term success of treatment, particularly where complex treatment is planned. Should the patient not respond adequately to advice, the treatment plan will need to be simplified.

A white spot enamel lesion on the buccal or lingual surface can be controlled by regular efficient removal of plaque; this approach is far preferable to operative intervention and will be successful where there is co-operation from the patient.

APPLICATION OF TOPICAL FLUORIDE

The application of fluoride solutions or, more recently, gels to the tooth surface as a method of reducing caries has been carried out since the 1940s. The effectiveness of the various solutions has been reviewed by Murray & Rugg-Gunn (1982). A number of well-controlled studies have shown only a small benefit from such applications and whilst the percentage reduction in caries might appear impressive, it is rarely more than one-third of a surface over a 3-year period and may not be clinically significant. To apply the topical fluoride, the teeth must first be thoroughly cleaned by the dentist or hygienist and dried, before application for 4 minutes of the solution with pledgets of cotton wool, or the gel in special trays. Both upper and lower teeth can be treated at once with the gel, whereas with the solution each jaw or each quadrant is usually treated separately. The fluoride gels taste unpleasant and have made some children feel sick. Applying fluoride is a procedure which is costly in time of professional personnel for small benefit; there are those who argue that time would be better spent concentrating on dietary advice. There is little value in applying fluoride solutions to teeth of people who have been brought up in areas with water fluoridation; if the patient has a caries problem, it is the diet which needs correction.

The most recent method of applying fluoride in the dental surgery has been to use a special varnish, Duraphat (Woelm Pharma GmbH, Eschwege, Germany), which is an alcoholic solution of resins containing 50 mg sodium fluoride per millilitre. The teeth should first be cleaned and dried, before the varnish is applied on a pledget of cotton wool. It is considerably quicker and more pleasant for the patient than fluoride gels. It is recommended that it is used twice a year and caries reduction from a number of surveys has been approximately 40% (Schmidt, 1981).

White spot lesions can be remineralized and prevented from demineralizing further by regular application of fluoride at low concentrations. The clinical effect is to harden the enamel surface even if discoloration remains. Microscopically, mineral is redeposited deep in the enamel. This may be achieved either with a low concentration fluoride mouthwash (0.05% NaF) or rubbing on fluoride toothpaste, applied daily. It must, of course, be accompanied by adequate control of diet and effective oral hygiene.

FISSURE SEALANTS

Fissures benefit least from water fluoridation and many are still liable to become carious in children who have always ingested fluoridated water. Even with the regular use of fluoride toothpaste, fissure caries may still occur and its detection is made more difficult by lack of early cavitation of enamel. Therefore, the application of a sealant to prevent a carious lesion developing in the fissures is of value. A resin sealant can be coated onto the enamel surface surrounding the fissure after it has been cleaned, isolated, conditioned and dried. Simonsen (1987) reported in a clinical trial that after 5 years sealant was completely lost from only 7% of the treated surfaces. After 10 years, sealant was completely present on 57%, partially present on 21% and caries or a restoration was present on 15%. When some of these patients were matched with patients who had not received sealants, the sealant group had caries or a restoration in 22% of surfaces whereas the non-sealant group had caries or a restoration in 68% of surfaces after 10 years.

As stated in the previous chapter, fissure caries occurs soon after tooth eruption and fissures that survive this period are unlikely to become carious. Therefore, to be an effective caries preventive measure, the sealant must be applied shortly after the tooth appears in the mouth when the tooth may be incompletely erupted. This may make adequate isolation of the tooth difficult, but isolation with rubber dam is most necessary to prevent moisture contamination which would interfere with successful retention of sealant. Plaque must be cleaned off the occlusal surface with pumice before the enamel on each side of the fissure is etched with a gel or solution (usually 35–50%) of phosphoric acid for 1 minute. The remaining acid and salts are then washed off with a waterspray for at least 15 seconds, and the tooth is dried thoroughly with compressed air before application of a dimethacrylate sealant resin which is polymerized by the application of intense light. Further details of resins will be covered in Chapter 7 and the acid-etch technique in Chapter 8.

Fissure sealants must be applied by suitably qualified personnel and so the cost of this preventive measure is high. However, used selectively to treat fissures at risk, this is a valuable way of preventing caries, particularly for patients with a high incidence of caries and low motivation.

It is not normally recommended that fissure sealants should be used to seal in caries that is known to extend into dentine, although two studies have reported that the lesions were arrested and most micro-organisms died out. The status of fissure sealants has been thoroughly reviewed by Silverstone (1982).

RESTORATIONS

The removal of caries from a cavity and insertion of a restoration can prevent further spread of caries and could therefore be considered a preventive measure. When a small restoration is combined with fissure sealing, the procedure is referred to as a preventive resin restoration. This restoration has gained clinical acceptance as a conservative method of treating early fissure caries and preventing its herthes spread. Use of this restoration should be accompanied by dietary counselling and a plague control programme.

Bibliography

Dowell T. B. & Joyston-Bechal S. (1981) Fluoride supplements — age related dosages. *British Dental Journal*, **150**, 273–275.

Greene J. C. & Vermillion J. R. (1960) The oral hygiene index: a method for classifying oral hygiene status. *Journal of the American Dental Association*, **61**, 172–179.

Gustafsson B. E., Quesnel C. E., Lanke L. S., Lundqvist C., Grahnen H., Bonow B. E. & Krasse B. (1954) The Vipeholm dental caries study. *Acta Odontologica Scandinavica*, **11**, 232–264.

Murray J. J. (1989) *The Prevention of Dental Disease*, 2nd edn. Oxford Medical Publications, Oxford.

Murray J. J. & Rugg-Gunn A. J. (1982) *Fluorides in Caries Prevention*, pp. 31–56, 100–126, 135–153. Wright, Bristol.

OPCS (1983) *Children's Dental Health 1983*. OPCS Monitor SS 83/2. HMSO, London. (Reprinted in *British Dental Journal*, **155**, 322–328.)

Schmidt H. F. M. (1981) Evaluation of Duraphat fluoride varnish as caries prophylactic based upon clinical results available in 1981. *Kariesprophylaxe*, **3**, 117–123.

Silverstone L. M. (1982) The use of pit and fissure sealants in dentistry, present status and future developments. *Pediatric Dentistry*, **4**, 16–21.

Silverstone L. M., Johnson N. W., Hardie J. M. & Williams R. A. D. (1981) *Dental Caries, Aetiology, Pathology and Prevention*, Part II, pp. 207–304. Macmillan, London.

Simonsen R. J. (1987) Retention and effectiveness of a single application of white sealant after 10 years. *Journal of the American Dental Association*, **115**, 31–36.

Todd J. E. (1975) *Children's Dental Health in England and Wales 1973*. HMSO, London.

Weaver R. (1944) Fluorosis and dental caries on Tyneside. *British Dental Journal*, **76**, 29–40.

3 Non-carious damage to teeth

3.1 Introduction

Non-carious damage to teeth is relatively much less common than dental caries and, with the exception of fractures which usually appear suddenly, is of slow onset. The conditions of attrition, abrasion and erosion are artificially divided, although they frequently appear in combination; they do not normally need treatment unless severe. However, by recognizing them at an early stage, measures can be instituted to prevent their becoming severe and avoid the need for treatment.

3.2 Fractures

Fractures may be caused by traumatic injuries, either direct blows to the teeth or indirectly by a blow to the mandible resulting in fracture of cusps, particularly of posterior teeth. In addition, severe occlusal pressures, particularly on teeth with large restorations and unprotected cusps, may also cause tooth fracture. The extent of fracture may range from crazed enamel through lost cusps to a split tooth which cannot be saved. Direct trauma most often affects upper anterior teeth, and because the blow strikes the labial surface of the teeth, cracks radiate backwards and are usually horizontal or oblique. With other fractures, forces are almost always applied to the occlusal surface, so the fracture lines are generally vertical.

Blows to anterior teeth most commonly affect sound teeth in children and, if left untreated, exposure of the wide dentinal tubules to dental plaque may lead to inflammation of the pulp, which must then be treated. On the other hand, posterior teeth which fracture under large occlusal pressures are normally heavily restored. In these teeth, few of the exposed dentinal tubules communicate with the pulp because of responses to the original caries and restorative procedures, i.e. tubular calcifications and extensive deposits of reactionary dentine in the pulp chamber; therefore, subsequent involvement of the pulp is less common.

Direct trauma may cause the following damage to one or more teeth:

1 Pulpal damage without fracture.
2 Crazing of enamel (infraction).
3 Fracture of enamel.

4 Fracture of enamel and dentine.
5 Fracture through the pulp.
6 Fracture of the crown extending into the root.
7 Intra-alveolar fracture of the root.
8 Extrusion, avulsion or intrusion.

PULPAL DAMAGE WITHOUT FRACTURE

A blow to the tooth may cause damage to the vessels where they pass through the apical foramen to supply the pulp, particularly in a tooth with a completely formed root. This may lead to degeneration or even death of the pulp, conditions which may not become apparent for some months. It is therefore necessary to observe these teeth and check pulpal vitality at regular intervals. It may be at least a year following trauma before the pulp responds again to vitality testing. Where evidence accumulates that the pulp has degenerated or died, root canal treatment is necessary to prevent an abscess occurring (for details see Chapters 5 and 14).

CRAZING OF ENAMEL (INFRACTION)

Crazing of enamel may be referred to as infraction of enamel. Crazed enamel itself rarely requires treatment, but the pulps of such teeth may degenerate or die because of damage at the time of injury to the vessels where they pass through the apical foramen or because of later bacterial invasion into dentine through the cracks in enamel. Again, where evidence accumulates that the pulp has degenerated, root canal treatment is necessary.

FRACTURE OF ENAMEL

If only a small amount of enamel has been lost, it may be most appropriate to carry out no restorative treatment. However, if the fractured edge is sharp or unsightly, it may be smoothed; loss of more enamel may require a restoration to be placed to improve appearance (for details see Chapters 8 and 9). The tooth should be observed subsequently in case the pulp degenerates.

FRACTURE OF ENAMEL AND DENTINE

Fracture through the dentine of a sound tooth opens up numerous tubules, the contents of which are extremely sensitive. The early placement of a restoration to cover the exposed tubules will relieve the pain; further, it prevents bacteria from invading the tubules and causing inflammation of the pulp. If a restoration is not placed, the bacterial invasion is likely to cause pulpal inflammation and eventual necrosis. A restoration will also restore the appearance of the patient's tooth, and it is usual to place a restoration in a tooth-coloured material, such as composite resin, which is retained by etched enamel. It should be placed immediately after the injury and fortunately it does not interfere with the subsequent regular checking of pulpal vitality. Should root canal treatment become necessary, access can easily be obtained through the palatal surface of the tooth.

FRACTURE THROUGH THE PULP

When the fracture involves the pulp in a mature tooth, it is necessary to remove the pulp, because efforts to keep it alive are often unsuccessful and the canal space is normally required for retention of an artificial crown to restore the shape of the tooth. Permanent restoration of the crown is performed after completion of root canal treatment; composite resin is suitable where loss of tooth structure is not extensive, otherwise a post crown is necessary (for details see Chapter 15).

In an immature tooth (Fig. 3.1), only part of the coronal pulp would be removed and a medicament of calcium hydroxide would then be placed over the pulpal surface to induce a hard tissue barrier. The purpose is to maintain pulpal vitality and allow the radicular pulp to continue root formation, after which root canal treatment could be carried out if required. The crown is normally restored with composite resin after the pulp has been treated.

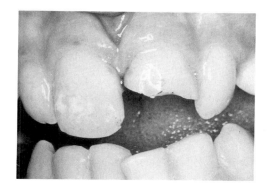

Fig. 3.1 The upper left cental incisor has a fractured incisal edge involving the pulp.

FRACTURE OF THE CROWN EXTENDING INTO THE ROOT

Where the fracture of the crown extends into the root, the broken piece of tooth may still remain in position when the patient attends for treatment because it is attached by periodontal fibres. The loose fragment should be removed under local anaesthesia so that the apical extent of fracture can be assessed. Where it is superficial to alveolar bone, the tooth may be restored after minor surgery to the gingivae (gingivoplasty) and root filling. Where it is deep to bone, restoration of the tooth is more difficult and has a less favourable prognosis because of the short length of remaining root. Also, it is more difficult to isolate the tooth to carry out root canal treatment, and extrusion of the root by orthodontic treatment would probably be required before the crown could be satisfactorily restored. Where the fracture is unfavourable, the remnants of the tooth are usually removed, and the tooth is replaced by a denture or bridge. However, it is preferable to retain the tooth where possible because of the disadvantages of these artificial replacements. In a few instances, removal of the tooth and closure of the space by orthodontic treatment may be considered.

INTRA-ALVEOLAR FRACTURE OF THE ROOT

The root may be fractured almost horizontally without the fracture communicating with the mouth; this is a closed intra-alveolar fracture. If the fracture site is close to the crown, the tooth has very little periodontal support, the prognosis is poor and the tooth may need to be extracted. The prognosis is much better where the fracture is close to the apex because of the greater periodontal attachment of the coronal fragment. Immediately following the injury, the fractured tooth must be splinted for 2 months to prevent excessive movement of the coronal fragment. With excessive movement the pulp could die, necessitating root canal treatment and jeopardizing the long-term prognosis. One of three outcomes may occur after splinting. The most favourable result is the uniting of the two parts of the root by hard tissue. Secondly, continued pulpal vitality of the coronal part without union is very acceptable, whilst thirdly, if pulpal necrosis occurs, its treatment by cleaning and filling of the root canal of the coronal part is preferable to extraction; the pulp in the apical part often remains vital and so can usually be left alone.

EXTRUSION, AVULSION OR INTRUSION

Where the tooth is partially displaced from its socket, i.e. extruded, it should be repositioned within minutes of the injury. The tooth should normally be splinted for 2 weeks and root canal treatment started about 10–14 days after trauma when any injuries to the periodontal tissues would have healed.

A tooth that has been completely knocked out, i.e. avulsed, can be repositioned, splinted and root treated in a similar way. The long-term prognosis is not so good, because the roots of many of these teeth may resorb, particularly if the tooth was out of the mouth for more than half an hour and had been allowed to dry out. Failure to carry out root treatment at the correct time may lead to extensive resorption.

A tooth that has been forced further into the alveolus, i.e. intruded, must, if it is to be retained, be repositioned orthodontically.

The reader should refer to a more comprehensive text (e.g.

Andreasen, 1981 and Andreasen & Andreasen, 1990) for further information on traumatic injuries.

OTHER FRACTURES

Severe occlusal pressures in heavily restored teeth can often lead to vertical cracks, especially in patients who grind their teeth. These cracks may be complete, in which case a cusp or side of tooth breaks away, or the split may extend into the root with the separate parts being loose but remaining in place. If there is no pulpal involvement the tooth may be restored most suitably with some form of extra-coronal restoration which holds together the weakened remains. If there is pulpal involvement, root canal treatment will be required first. Where the crack passes through the root furcation, extraction is normally the only treatment.

Alternatively, the crack may be incomplete with no detectable movement of the cusps; however, on biting, the patient can elicit sharp pain of short duration. Careful examination of the tooth, particularly with an intraoral light, will usually reveal hairline cracks. This condition is given the name, cracked tooth syndrome. Where the crack is incomplete, the usual treatment is to construct a restoration which onlays the occlusal surface to spread the load and to hold the parts together.

3.3 Attrition

Whenever teeth make contact, they wear, and the more often that they make contact the greater is the wear. It is therefore usual to find some wear of the occlusal and approximal surfaces of teeth that have been present in the mouth for a number of years. This wear caused by tooth contact is called attrition. Since enamel is so hard and opposing teeth make contact infrequently because they are lubricated by saliva, wear is normally very limited even after several decades.

Mild wear may often be observed as the formation of a facet on the tips of the canine teeth and the loss of the tubercles on incisal edges. Such a condition requires no intervention by the dentist.

Further wear will expose dentine, and the pulp responds by tubular calcification in the affected exposed area and by the formation of reactionary dentine. Wear caused by a grinding habit alone causes even wear of dentine and enamel. Where a shallow saucer-shaped depression bounded by a ring of enamel is created, there is usually erosion superimposed on attrition (Fig 3.2). In its early stages, observation and advice on diet is best because the cavity is not amenable to filling.

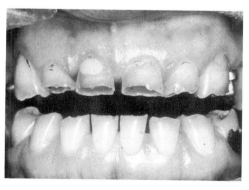

Fig. 3.2 Marked attrition with superimposed erosion of the upper incisors with less affecting the lower incisors. The patient had few remaining posterior teeth.

Occasionally, however, teeth show excessive wear. Very often this has been caused by a subconscious grinding habit of the patient, particularly at night when there is little saliva to act as lubricant. When wear becomes extensive, a considerable amount of the clinical crown may be lost, and if the rate of wear exceeds the rate of deposition of reactionary dentine, the pulp could become exposed and necessitate root canal treatment. Intervention is necessary when wear becomes unsightly, the pulp is in danger of exposure or the occlusion becomes substantially altered. A veneer crown is frequently required and whilst one in cast gold is suitable for posterior teeth, a metal–ceramic crown must be used on anteriors to combine appearance with strength. Wear normally affects a large number of teeth and therefore treatment is inevitably extensive. It is difficult and time-consuming because the patient's occlusion frequently has to be reconstructed; this treatment is unsuitable for the inexperienced operator.

3.4 Abrasion

This is wear of the teeth not caused by tooth contact; such causes are over-zealous horizontal toothbrushing with abrasive toothpaste or wearing of an incisal edge by objects such as hairgrips or smokers' pipes.

The pulp responds to exposed dentine by tubular calcification and reactionary dentine. The exposed dentine is rarely sensitive and this condition is most often found as a V-shaped groove close to the gingival margin. There is frequently gingival recession as a result of the excessive brushing but the gingivae are usually healthy. This condition should become less widespread as the abrasivity of most toothpastes has now been reduced.

Treatment should consist of advising the patient to use an alternative, less destructive toothbrushing technique with a less abrasive toothpaste, or to discontinue the biting habit. In the mild form of the condition it is preferable to observe the cavity. Where the groove gingivally is very deep and the pulp endangered, it is sensible to fill the cavity with an adhesive cement; this is a non-invasive procedure and details are described in Chapters 8 and 9.

3.5 Erosion

This is loss of mineral by acid erosion. It is usually caused by an acid diet, such as drinking large amounts of citrus juices or fizzy drinks, eating large numbers of oranges or sharp apples, or a great deal of yoghurt. It may also be caused by regurgitation of acid from the stomach in patients with digestive disorders, such as hiatus hernia, or in patients suffering from anorexia nervosa or bulimia nervosa.

Erosion from industrial fumes has occurred, but these should cease to be a continuing source in view of Health and Safety at Work regulations.

Regular repeated applications of weak acids to the surfaces of teeth remove mineral. In many patients, tooth loss by erosion is accelerated by accompanying attrition and abrasion. The brushing of teeth after the application of acid significantly increases loss of tooth substance. Normally a number of teeth are affected on similar surfaces while other surfaces of these teeth may be completely unaffected. In dietary erosion, the buccal surfaces of the upper teeth (Fig. 3.3) and occlusal surfaces of the lower teeth are most affected. Regurgitation erosion is most severe on the palatal surfaces of the upper anterior teeth (Fig. 3.4). In the early stage, perikymata on the tooth surface disappear and the tooth has a characteristic flat appearance, but the enamel has a normal colour as opposed to the chalkiness in caries. Further erosion exposes dentine, which is often sensitive as the acid demineralizes the tubular calcifications. Eventually the pulp may become inflamed.

The cause of the erosion may be difficult to establish and require taking a detailed history. Where there is an associated medical condition, the patient's doctor should be involved. Treatment of dietary erosion should consist of dietary analysis and dissuading the patient from excessive intake of citrus fruit and other low pH food and drink. Where only enamel has been affected the teeth are best observed, but where there is dentine involvement and the teeth are unsightly and sensitive the labial surfaces may be restored with a restorative material retained on etched enamel at the periphery (Fig. 3.3). More extensive loss, particularly where occluding surfaces are involved, may require the construction of veneer crowns.

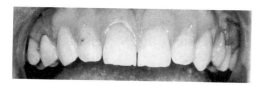

Fig. 3.3 *Top*: dietary erosion affecting the upper central incisors. *Bottom*: after restoration of the defects with composite resin.

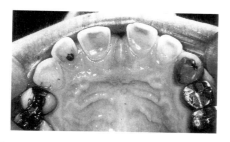

Fig. 3.4 Typical appearance of regurgitation erosion which has affected the palatal surfaces of the upper anterior teeth.

Bibliography

Andreasen J. O. (1981) *Traumatic Injuries of the Teeth*, 2nd edn. Munksgaard, Copenhagen.

Andreasen J. O. & Andreasen F. M (1990) *Essentials of Traumatic Injuries to the Teeth*. Munksgaard, Copenhagen.

Cameron C. E. (1976) The cracked tooth syndrome: additional findings. *Journal of the American Dental Association*, **93**, 971–975.

Eccles J. D. (1979) Dental erosion of non-industrial origin. A clinical survey and classification. *Journal of Prosthetic Dentistry*, **42**, 649–653.

Smith B. G. N. & Knight J. K. (1984) A comparison of patterns of tooth wear with aetiological factors. *British Dental Journal*, **157**, 16–19.

4 Instruments

4.1 Introduction

Before considering cavity preparation, the reader should be aware of the instruments at his disposal so that the most suitable one can be used; also, it is all too easy to draw diagrams of preparations which are impractical. The operator will be governed by his instruments, although they should never be made the scapegoat for poor technique or incorrect choice; small cavities require small instruments both for preparation and for restoration.

A major problem of working in the mouth is restricted access, both visual and physical. It is substantially alleviated by the working end of most instruments being set at an angle to the handle (Fig. 4.1). However, the active tip of the instrument is positioned very close to the long axis of the handle, allowing good control by the operator. If the tip were away from the long axis, the operator would have poor control of the instrument, which consequently would be liable to slip. Instruments which have their shaft bent to bring the active tip back into the long axis are called contra-angle and are the most widely used. Straight instruments are the most efficient but are of limited use in the mouth; however, they are preferable where access ceases to be a problem, e.g. working in the laboratory.

Instruments can be divided into two broad categories, rotary and hand; as in so many other aspects of life, mechanized instruments are used when and wherever possible, unless they are unsuitable. Most operative procedures on teeth are carried out with rotary instruments,

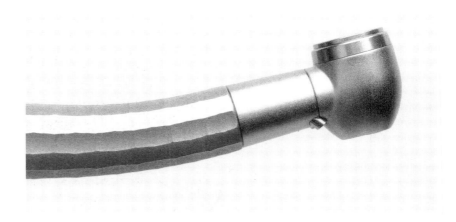

Fig. 4.1 Turbine handpiece with its head set an angle to the shaft bringing the cutting tip close to the long axis of the handle.

so these will be considered first. The selection of particular instruments for the various procedures will be covered in subsequent chapters.

4.2 Rotary instruments

These may be divided into two groups: high-speed and low-speed instruments. The high-speed instruments are used for removing hard tooth substance and old restorations, while the low-speed instruments are principally used for removing carious dentine, refining, finishing and polishing.

HIGH-SPEED INSTRUMENTS

The high-speed instrument is an air-driven turbine (Fig. 4.1) and is universally used for cavity preparation because it rapidly removes enamel, dentine and restorative materials without effort. The patient finds it acceptable because tooth preparation is quick and vibration-free. The basic design of these instruments has not changed since their introduction by Borden in the late 1950s. The handpiece is attached to a flexible hose which supplies compressed air to operate the turbine. The handle of the instrument is a metal tube and is shaped to be convenient to hold. The working head of the handpiece, which is always contra-angled, contains the turbine. At each end of the turbine is a bearing, usually a ball-bearing but some were manufactured with an air-bearing. The cutting instrument, known as a bur, which has a shank of specified diameter and length, fits into a chuck in the turbine; the bur is usually retained by friction although some manufacturers provide a chuck which needs to be tightened with a key. Recently, several manufacturers have produced push-button chucks which allow easier placement and removal of burs; there is also less risk of damaging the burs or accidental injury to the person changing the bur. Handpieces are delicate and serious damage may occur if they are accidently dropped. It is now common for manufacturers to include a light guide in the head of the handpiece to allow the operator to see better (Fig. 4.2), the light bulb being in the end of the turbine hose. Because the bur revolves at high speed, its tip would rapidly overheat the tooth unless coolant was used, so the base of the handpiece head contains one or more apertures (Fig. 4.2) which allow a spray of water mixed with air to play on the cutting tip. The turbine is operated by a footswitch. The speed of the turbine is dependent on the exact type, but is usually in the range of 250 000–450 000 r.p.m. The present generation of turbine handpiece operates near the lower end of

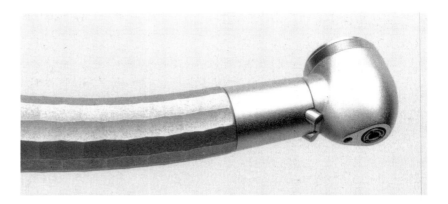

Fig. 4.2 The head of the turbine handpiece is tapered for good vision. At the base of the head is an aperture for the waterspray to cool the bur tip, and two light guides.

this speed range, has a large turbine for power and has a tapered head to increase visibility of the bur tip.

During operation it is essential that an adequate volume of spray is used to prevent overheating at the bur tip and, furthermore, the spray must not become obstructed by cusps while a cavity in a tooth is being deepened. The visibility for the operator is reduced by the waterspray but no cavity must be prepared without it. An advantage of the waterspray is that it washes all the debris out of the cavity and allows continuous working. Concurrently, the water is removed from the operating field by high volume suction.

A sharp revolving bur cuts both enamel and dentine rapidly when held against the tooth. The application of pressure is unnecessary and undesirable as it could lead to overcutting, overheating or stalling; stalling occurs particularly with older types of turbine and those with

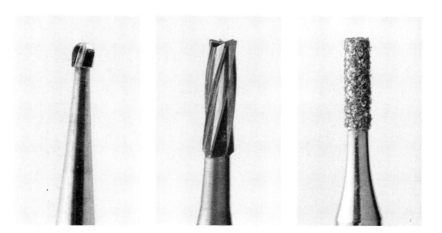

Fig. 4.3 Burs for use in the turbine handpiece. *Left*: a round tungsten carbide bur. *Middle*: a parallel-sided fissure tungsten carbide bur. *Right*: a parallel-sided fissure diamond bur.

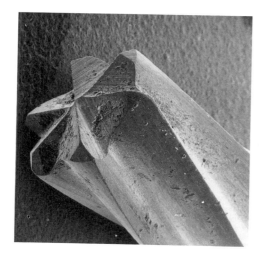

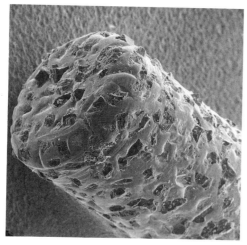

Fig. 4.4 Scanning electron micrographs of the tip of a fissure tungsten carbide bur (*top*) and a fissure diamond bur (*bottom*).

air-bearings. Turbine burs are of two basic shapes: a spherical cutting tip, usually known as a round bur; and a cylindrical tip, usually known as a fissure bur (Fig. 4.3). The round bur is widely used to prepare small cavities and create special features in large cavities; it cuts well on both its end and its side. For larger cavities and extracoronal preparations, a fissure bur is used; it may be parallel-sided or tapered, and may have a flat or round end. Extensive use is made of the fissure bur's ability to cut on its side, although most fissure burs will also cut well on their end (Fig. 4.4). A bur which combines the attributes of both is pear-shaped (Fig. 4.5).

The cutting part of a turbine bur is made from tungsten carbide or diamond particles. Both types are widely used for intracoronal preparations, but for extracoronal preparations diamond burs are more appropriate as they are less brittle in long thin shapes.

Tungsten carbide burs are manufactured by brazing a tungsten carbide/cobalt composite tip onto a steel shank before the cutting flutes are ground into the tip. When new, these burs cut extremely efficiently, but they eventually become blunt; their life can be measured in tens of cavities. When the bur becomes blunt it fails to cut the tooth efficiently and should be discarded. Tungsten carbide burs usually have blades with a continuous edge (Fig. 4.3); these are called plain-cut and they do leave a very smooth surface to the tooth. It is advisable for the operator and dental surgery assistant (DSA) to wear eye protection when drilling out old amalgam restorations as these burs may cause large pieces of material to fly off; also, the tips of burs which have been bent may separate when rotated in the turbine, producing a dangerous projectile. Cast metal alloys (e.g. gold) are only readily drilled with a sharp new tungsten carbide round bur or the more recently introduced bur with fine serrations in the blades (Fig. 4.6); eye protection is essential for the operator and DSA as the head of the round bur is liable to snap off during the drilling of these alloys; the tooth should also be isolated to prevent the possibility of the patient inhaling the bur tip.

Tungsten carbide fissure burs may have blades which have coarse serrations in the cutting edge; these are known as cross-cut burs and are not widely used in the turbine handpiece because of the rough surface that they leave on the tooth. Some tungsten carbide burs are produced with multiple flutes (Fig. 4.7); these are less efficient at removing large amounts of tooth substance but are most suitable for finishing preparations and the surface of restorations. The concept of multiple flutes may be taken *ad infinitum*, in which case one is left with a tungsten carbide blank; this is a useful bur for smoothing cavity margins and is named 'Baker–Curson' after its originators (Fig. 4.7).

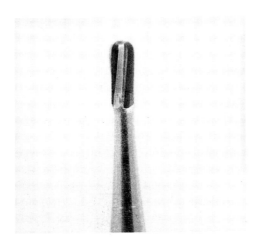

Fig. 4.5 A pear-shaped tungsten carbide bur for use in the turbine handpiece.

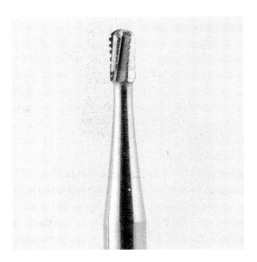

Fig. 4.6 A fine serrated pear-shaped tungsten carbide bur, particularly effective at cutting metal for use in the turbine handpiece.

Tungsten carbide burs are unsuitable for cutting composite resin as this material blunts them quite rapidly.

Diamond burs consist of graded particles of industrial diamond held on a blank steel shaft by an electro-deposited metal film. The cutting efficiency of these burs is dependent on the ground tooth particles being washed off the surface of the bur by the waterspray; and their life is longer than that of tungsten carbide burs. The coarseness of the diamond particles governs their use; the standard burs (see Figs 4.3 & 4.4) have a coarse grit which leaves a rough surface on the tooth but enables rapid tooth preparation. Finer grit burs are used to give a smooth surface to a preparation created with coarse burs, but general tooth preparation is not undertaken with fine grit burs because it would take too long. Diamond burs are suitable for removing old restorations of amalgam or composite resin. Diamond burs will cut through porcelain whereas tungsten carbide burs will blunt rapidly. However, diamond burs are ineffective in cutting through cast metal alloys; in contrast, the finely serrated tungsten carbide burs are very efficient. Because diamond burs are widely used for extracoronal preparations they are consequently produced in an extensive range of shapes.

Turbine burs have shanks 1.6 mm in diameter (1/16 inch) and are usually 19 mm in length (3/4 inch). For extracoronal preparation some of the burs are longer to facilitate tooth preparation; but for most cavity preparation, access is restricted with a long bur, as the head of the turbine hits the opposing teeth and the extra length of cutting surface may cause damage to another part of the tooth. The diameter of the cutting tip is never large, first because it is unnecessary as a small bur revolving so fast can remove tooth substance rapidly, and secondly because a large tip rotating at speed would strain the turbine bearings and chuck. Large burs in a friction-grip chuck could come out and this would be dangerous.

LOW-SPEED INSTRUMENTS

Low-speed instrumentation has been available for considerably longer than air turbine handpieces, but is not now routinely used for most cavity preparation as it takes considerably longer and more effort is involved. The hardness of enamel is not always appreciated by the modern operator, who may not have prepared a large cavity entirely with low-speed instruments.

Low-speed instruments are used for procedures such as excavating carious dentine, refining retentive grooves in cavities, finishing cavities and restorations, and polishing.

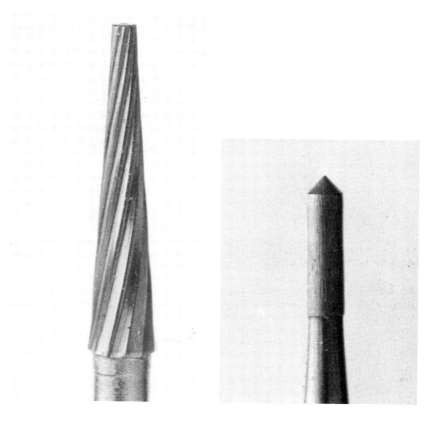

Fig. 4.7 Tungsten carbide finishing burs for use in the turbine handpiece. *Left*: a long tapered multibladed bur. *Right*: a Baker–Curson bur which has no blades.

Low-speed handpieces are available in contra-angle form (Fig. 4.8) and in straight form; the latter is rarely used in the mouth because of limited access, but is also produced in a more robust form for use in the dental laboratory. The principles of design of these handpieces have changed little over many years. The handle of the instrument is a

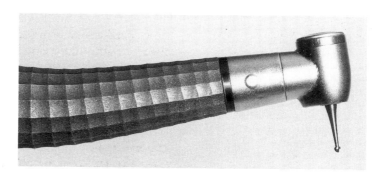

Fig. 4.8 A round bur in a contra-angle low-speed handpiece.

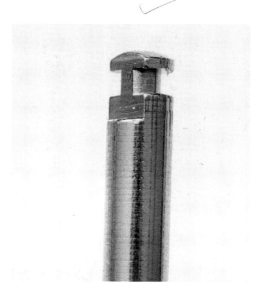

Fig. 4.9 The non-working end of a bur for the contra-angle low-speed handpiece showing a flattened face and groove which engage into the drive gear.

metal sleeve which fits over a drive shaft, which is extended to the head of a contra-angle handpiece by gears. The drive to the base of the handpiece is now usually provided by a small air or electric motor on a flexible hose, whereas it used to be by a pulley-guided cord attached to a large engine on the dental unit. The operator has gained increased flexibility but often less control of bur speed. Modern low-speed handpieces have built-in watersprays and light guides.

The bur is held in the head of a contra-angle handpiece by either a latch-joint or occasionally a friction-grip chuck. The end of the bur has a flattened face to engage the drive gear and a latch seats in a groove on the bur to prevent it from falling out of the handpiece (Fig. 4.9).

The speed of the bur is variable in the range 0–40 000 r.p.m., although only electric motors can work at the top speeds. At any but the lowest speeds, waterspray is essential, but it is only within the last few years that watersprays have been manufactured as an integral part of the low-speed handpiece. The operation of the handpiece is controlled by a footswitch; the speed of electric motors may be varied by the foot control but with air motors it must usually be preselected prior to use.

A low-speed handpiece is used in quite a different way from a turbine handpiece; a more powerful force is used to rotate the bur, which is often larger, at low speed. Therefore, the operator needs more effort to hold the handpiece steady; otherwise the bur tends to bite into the tooth and move the drill to cut part of the tooth that was not intended. The drilling of hard tooth substance requires the application of pressure by the operator, whereas carious dentine is removed almost passively, mainly by holding the handpiece steady. Bur shanks are of a larger diameter, 2.35 mm (3/32 inch), than those for a turbine handpiece, and standard burs for the contra-angle low-speed handpiece are also longer, 22 mm (7/8 inch). The range of cutting tips of the burs extends to larger sizes than turbine burs. For most straight handpieces, even longer burs are used.

The majority of burs for low-speed handpieces are made of hardened steel, which is not corrosion-resistant, because manufacturers have been accustomed to producing them at low cost and they were in use before the development of diamond and tungsten carbide burs. Steel burs have a short working life, become blunted rapidly by enamel and will rust. Some burs are now made in stainless steel.

Steel burs for cavity preparation are available in several basic shapes (Fig. 4.10). The round-headed bur, which is frequently referred to as a 'rose-head', is used particularly in the larger sizes for removal of carious dentine and in the smaller sizes for refining retentive grooves in cavities. The design of the bur tip allows the bur to cut effectively with its

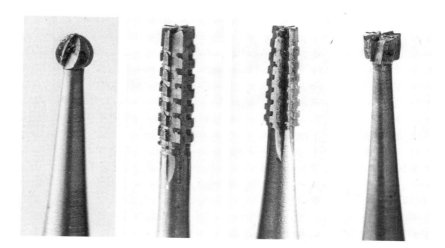

Fig. 4.10 Several basic shapes of steel bur for use in the low-speed handpiece. *Left*: a round bur. *Second from left*: a flat fissure bur. *Second from right*: a tapered fissure bur. *Right*: an inverted cone bur.

tip (Fig. 4.11). The flat fissure bur is a parallel-sided milling bur, usually cross-cut to increase efficiency; it will also cut with its end but this is not as effective as using its side. At one time this bur in the low-speed handpiece was the main instrument for cavity preparation before it was displaced by the turbine handpiece. The tapered fissure bur is, as its name suggests, used for tapered preparations, originally as the main bur for inlay preparations, but more recently it has only been used for refinements such as grooves. The inverted cone bur is widest at its tip and this made it popular for placing retentive grooves into the walls of cavities by lateral movement. In some circumstances these burs can extend a cavity inadvertently close to the pulp, and they are not now widely used. An end-cutting bur (Fig. 4.12) is intended to cut only with its end. Therefore, it is a relatively inefficient bur, because debris is not easily cleared from its blades. Through a lack of any side-cutting ability it is liable to introduce irregular steps into the floor of the preparation, and is not often used.

All these burs are available in a range of sizes which are numbered according to the diameter of the cutting tip. Often, the previously used British size number accompanies the International Organization for Standardization (ISO) number on packets of burs. Table 4.1 lists the conversion between the two systems for the smaller sizes of bur. In the United States, different numbering systems are used.

In addition to burs for cavity preparation, a range of multifluted steel burs are produced for finishing preparations and restorations (Fig. 4.12).

Diamond and tungsten carbide burs are also produced for the low-speed handpiece, but in a more restricted range than for turbine handpieces.

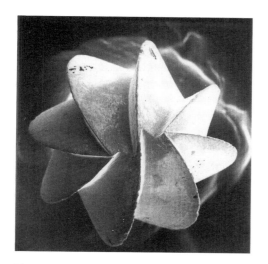

Fig. 4.11 A scanning electron micrograph of the tip of a round steel bur for use in the low-speed handpiece.

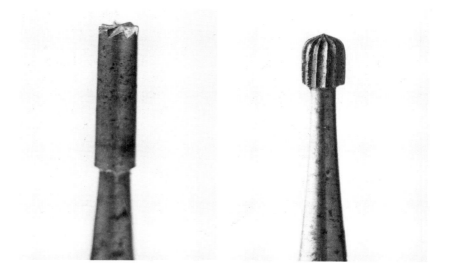

Fig. 4.12 An end-cutting steel bur (*left*) which is intended to cut with its end; it lacks side-cutting ability. A pear-shaped steel finishing bur (*right*). Both burs are used in the low-speed handpiece.

For many years, a series of mounted abrasive stones in a variety of shapes and materials has been available. These stones may be used to grind enamel, dentine and restorations. In more recent years, mounted abrasive rubber points have become available for smoothing the surfaces of restorations. Their abrasivity is dependent on the type and size of the particles incorporated.

There is a great range of wheel stones and discs made from a variety of materials which can be mounted onto mandrels (Fig. 4.13). The majority use the screw mandrel, whereas flexible discs tend to be used with a snap-on mandrel (Moore's) because they can be changed more easily (Fig. 4.14). Apart from the flexible discs which may be used to trim the accessible parts of restorations on anterior teeth, the major use of these wheels and discs is in the laboratory.

Brushes are produced in different sizes of cup and wheel form (Fig.

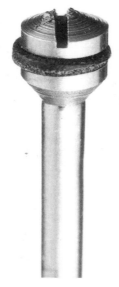

Fig. 4.13 The head of a screw mandrel for mounting abrasive stones or discs.

Table 4.1 The relation between the numbering systems for the smaller sizes of burs.*

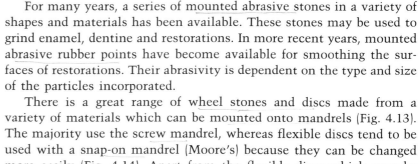

ISO (0.1 mm)	006	008	010	012	014	016	018	021
UK	½	1	2	3	4	5	6	7
UK and US (tapered fissure)	–	699	700	701	–	702	–	703
UK and US (pear shape)	–	330	331	332	333	–	–	–

* Bur sizes are determined by the maximum diameter of the cutting head.

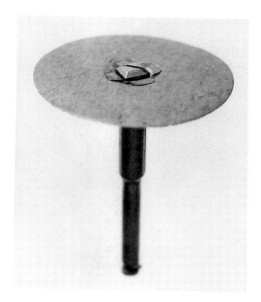

Fig. 4.14 A metal-centred abrasive disc on a Moore's mandrel for use in the low-speed handpiece.

4.15) in both natural bristle and nylon. The smallest cup form is used for polishing restorations intraorally, whereas the others are used in the laboratory for polishing cast restorations.

Low-speed handpieces usually have interchangeable heads which may reduce bur speed or increase bur speed; speed-increasing heads only accept turbine burs since bur speeds may be as high as 160 000 r.p.m. A smaller head (often called a miniature head or children's head) for use with shorter low-speed burs is useful when access is restricted, e.g. in children. Also, a head with sealed bearings is produced for polishing procedures to prevent abrasive particles entering and damaging the mechanism.

4.3 Hand instruments

Many of these instruments were developed before the widespread use of rotary instruments; therefore, there is a great variety but few operators now use an extensive range. They will be considered by their use.

INSTRUMENTS FOR EXAMINATION

Mirror

The dental mirror (Fig. 4.16) has a small circular mirror head attached to a handle. It allows the operator to observe the distal aspects of

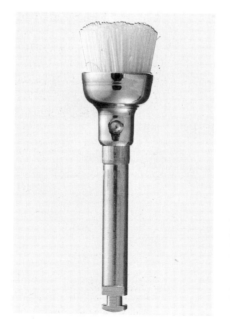

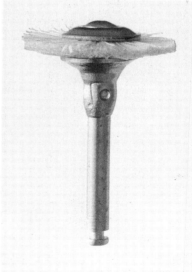

Fig. 4.15 Brushes for use in the low-speed handpiece. *Left*: a small cup. *Right*: in wheel form.

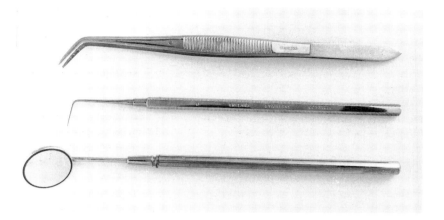

Fig. 4.16 Instruments for examination. *Top*: college tweezers. *Middle*: probe. *Bottom*: mirror.

teeth, is a useful retractor of the cheek or tongue and is often used simply to reflect light onto the teeth. The mirror is normally plane surfaced; a front-surfaced mirror is more valuable than a rear-surfaced one as the image is sharp; however, the consequences of scratching the surface are more serious. The inexperienced operator may initially find difficulty in working with a mirror as movements are reversed.

Probe

The most widely used probe is right-angled with a sharp point (Fig. 4.16). It is used for exploring the integrity of the surfaces of teeth and margins of restorations. It is also used to assess the hardness of dentine during cavity preparation in the treatment of caries. For the detection of caries on the approximal surface, a short hooked probe, usually double-ended (Briault), is used. The tip of the probe is tempered steel, and should not therefore be heated otherwise it would become soft and bend in use.

Probes may be used to measure the depth of periodontal pockets; for this, a special probe with a blunt end and graduated millimetre scale is used to assess pocket depth accurately (Fig. 4.17).

Tweezers

College tweezers (Fig. 4.16) have serrated beaks set at an angle to the handle. They are used to hold pledgets of cotton wool and to convey small items to and from the operating field. Tweezers are also available in locking form and these have the advantage of holding the

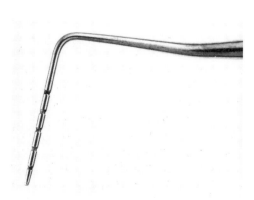

Fig. 4.17 The tip of a periodontal probe with graduated markings.

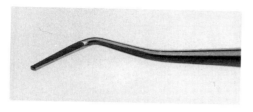

Fig. 4.18 A binangled chisel with the cutting blade close to the long axis of the handle.

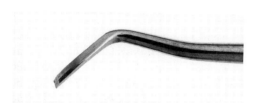

Fig. 4.19 A gingival margin trimmer with an angled blade (1 mm wide).

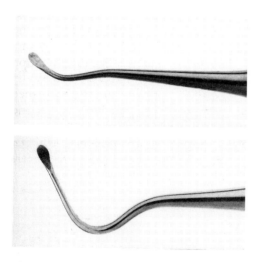

Fig. 4.20 *Top*: a widely used excavator with its tip close to the long axis of the handle. *Bottom*: a long-bladed excavator.

small pledget, pin or root filling point in the tweezers for as long as required.

INSTRUMENTS FOR TOOTH PREPARATION

Chisels

These are essentially scaled-down versions of a carpenter's chisel. The straight chisel is of limited use in the mouth but the contra-angled chisel (Fig. 4.18) with its cutting tip set at an angle to the handle and close to its long axis is used to finish enamel margins of cavities. Several different versions of the contra-angled chisel are available to suit the different margins of a cavity; those with the blade in the same plane as the angled shaft are called hatchet chisels, while those with the blade at right angles are called binangled chisels. The chisel is used to plane away unsupported enamel after cavity preparation with rotary instruments, and should be used even where the cavity has been prepared with tungsten carbide burs because unsupported enamel prisms may still remain.

A modified chisel, the gingival margin trimmer, is used to trim the enamel margins on the gingival wall of an approximal cavity in a posterior tooth (Fig. 4.19). The cutting edge is set at an angle to the curved blade to facilitate trimming of the enamel margin. The instruments are double-ended and come in pairs: one instrument for the mesial and the other for the distal. The width of the blade is in the range 1:0–1.5 mm; the narrow blades are suitable for small cavities but are more difficult to control in large cavities. The blade shown in Fig. 4.19 is 1.0 mm wide.

Excavators

These can be considered as small shovels with a sharp edge; they were designed to dig out carious dentine in a controlled manner because the shape of their cutting edge prevents deep penetration, in a similar way to using a chisel on its bevel. Excavators are also extensively used for shaping and trimming soft restorative materials. The cutting blade may be disc- or pear-shaped (Fig. 4.20); the pear-shaped blade is considered to survive more resharpening. The most widely used excavator is contra-angled with its blade close to the axis of the handle for good control. For the very small cavity a smaller excavator is more convenient, whereas for the occasional deep cavity a long-bladed excavator is necessary (Fig. 4.20), but neither variant is suitable for routine use.

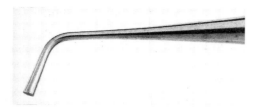

Fig. 4.21 An amalgam plugger with a smooth flat end.

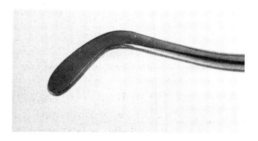

Fig. 4.22 A flat-bladed instrument used for placing plastic restorative materials hence the name 'flat plastic'.

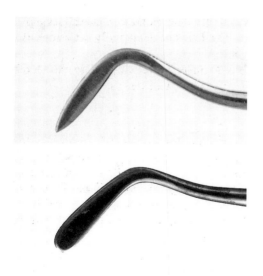

Fig. 4.23 Carvers: *Top:* ½ Hollenbach. *Bottom:* Ward's No. 2.

Excavators are double-ended to enable their use with a left- or right-handed sweep.

INSTRUMENTS FOR PLACING AND SHAPING MATERIALS

Pluggers

These are usually small cylinders used to compress restorative materials, principally amalgam, into a prepared cavity. The head has a flat end and the smaller it is, the greater the pressure that can be applied to compress the material (Fig. 4.21). Most of these instruments are double-ended with one end larger than the other. Pluggers used for amalgam now have smooth flat ends to avoid clogging, whereas in the days of hand-mixed amalgam serrated pluggers were used to control placement of material.

Plastics

These are flat-bladed instruments (Fig. 4.22) used for placing restorative materials in a soft deformable state, such as anterior filling materials, linings and temporary fillings, hence the name 'flat plastic'. The instruments are usually double-ended with one blade axially rotated at right angles to the other. The blade is blunt and is unsuitable for carving materials such as amalgam. The majority of these instruments are made from stainless steel; however, manufacturers have recently provided special coatings on the working tip to stop restorative materials sticking to them. In some cases the instrument has been teflon-coated and in others a ceramic coating has been applied. These coatings may be damaged by rough cleaning or when immersed in an ultrasonic bath.

Carvers

These instruments have a sharp blade as they are intended for carving soft materials, e.g. amalgam before it has hardened or inlay wax after it has hardened. They are usually double-ended and have been manufactured in several designs; two widely used instruments (1/2 Hollenbach and Ward's No. 2) are shown in Fig. 4.23.

Burnishers

These are similar to pluggers but have a rounded end instead of a flat one (Fig. 4.24). They are intended for adapting the fine margins of cast gold restorations and for contouring soft materials such as temporary fillings, partially set linings or amalgam prior to carving; they may

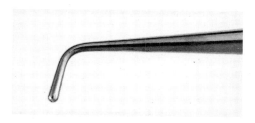

Fig. 4.24 A pear-shaped burnisher.

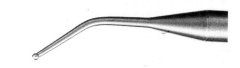

Fig. 4.25 A lining applicator.

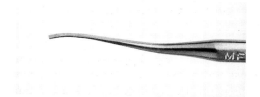

Fig. 4.26 A watch spring scaler.

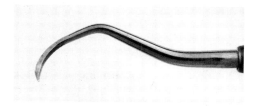

Fig. 4.27 A sickle scaler.

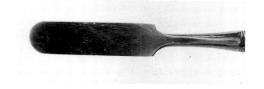

Fig. 4.28 A spatula.

also be used to give a smooth surface to carved amalgam. Burnishers are suitable for applying fluid-consistency lining materals to large cavities; in small cavities a special lining applicator (Fig. 4.25) is best.

Scalers

These instruments are primarily intended for removing deposits of calculus from the surfaces of teeth. Two types of scaler are useful in operative dentistry: the watch spring scaler and the sickle scaler.

The watch spring scaler (Fig. 4.26), also called a push scaler or periodontal chisel, is used to remove easily accessible deposits of supragingival calculus from the approximal surfaces of lower anterior teeth. It may also be used as a fine enamel chisel, particularly where an adjacent tooth restricts access to a conventional chisel which is thicker.

The sickle scaler (Fig. 4.27) has a fine pointed blade which has two cutting edges and is usually curved. Its small size allows good interproximal penetration and it is suitable for removing supragingival calculus and shallow deposits of subgingival calculus. It may also be used to carve the gingival aspect of partially set restorative materials such as amalgam and glass ionomer cement.

The curette is similar to a sickle but has a rounded tip and a rounded base to the blade; in cross-section it is semicircular as opposed to the triangular shape of a sickle. It is mainly used for removing supragingival and subgingival calculus on posterior teeth. Again, it may also be used to carve the gingival aspect of partially set restorative materials.

The periodontal hoe has a small blade at right angles to the shank. It is used for removing subgingival calculus in deep pockets.

Spatulas

These are instruments with a large blade used for mixing dental materials. Those for mixing lining cements are made of stainless steel (Fig. 4.28). Spatulas with harder blades of stellite (Co–Cr) or agate are recommended for mixing glass-based cements, such as glass ionomer or silicate. Non-metallic spatulas are advised for mixing some composite resins; they are usually disposable and supplied with the restorative material by the manufacturer.

MATERIALS USED FOR HAND INSTRUMENTS

The working tips of most instruments are made from stainless steel because of their strength and resistance to corrosion; carbon steel is now no longer used because of its susceptibility to corrosion. The instrument handle may be formed from the same piece of stainless steel as the working tip or may be of a different material, such as chromium-plated brass, aluminium alloy or ceramic. All these materials resist corrosion during sterilization in an autoclave, although aluminium alloys must not be placed in alkaline solutions. Aluminium alloy handles have two advantages over stainless steel handles; first, their size may be increased to improve control while they still feel light to hold; secondly, the manufacturers have the ability to colour them to enable ready identification according to usage. Handles are usually serrated to increase grip in the operator's hand. Instruments with round handles, compared with hexagonal ones, are more likely to roll off the bracket table onto the floor or patient.

4.4 3-in-1 syringe

The 3-in-1 syringe has become an indispensible piece of modern dental equipment. It is attached to the end of a flexible hose, which carries compressed air and water. There is a single nozzle and two depressible buttons (Fig. 4.29). Depression of one produces a jet of compressed air, depression of the other produces a jet of water, while depression of both together produces a spray. By varying the pressure on the buttons the intensity can be altered. The syringe is used to wash away debris and to dry teeth. Some manufacturers have produced these syringes with heaters to deliver air and water at body temperature. However, this has been discontinued to prevent the syringe being a breeding ground for bacteria in the water supply.

4.5 Aspirators

It is necessary to remove water which has been introduced to the operating field by rotary instruments and the 3-in-1 syringe. This is achieved by high volume suction, with a large bore aspirator, a small bore aspirator or a saliva ejector (Fig. 4.30) attached to a flexible hose.

The large bore aspirator will efficiently remove the large volume of water produced by a turbine handpiece; it is usually held by the DSA and significantly improves the ease of working. The aspirator may also be used as a retractor of the cheek or tongue. The saliva ejector, being flexible, can be bent to allow its tip to suck water out of the floor of the mouth. The saliva ejector without its tip is valuable for collecting excess restorative material during carving of restorations.

Should the aspirator inadvertently consume a dental restoration,

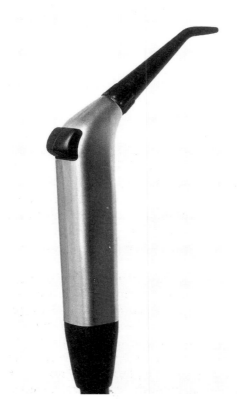

Fig. 4.29 A 3-in-1 syringe with a single nozzle and two depressible buttons; at its base it is attached to a flexible hose.

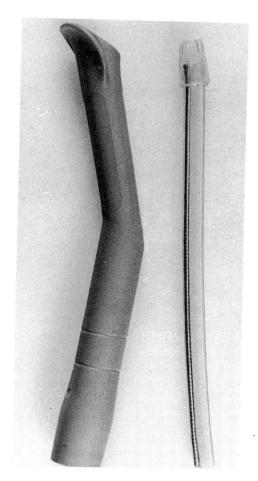

Fig. 4.30 A wide bore aspirator (*left*) and a disposable flexible saliva ejector (*right*).

there is a filter inside the dental unit from which the restoration may be retrieved.

4.6 Maintenance

Instruments will give many years of service if they are carefully maintained. They should only be used for their intended purpose; misuse will lead to strain and wear or breakage.

Handpieces should be cleaned after use and lubricated as recommended by the manufacturer. This will substantially prolong their life. Should a bearing show wear, then its return to the manufacturer for repair will prevent more serious damage occurring.

Hand instruments should not be dropped on the floor, because if one fell on its working end, it invariably would become bent and liable to subsequent fracture. Instruments should not be heated in an open flame as this will reduce their strength and they will subsequently bend in normal use very easily.

Chisels, excavators and scalers require periodic sharpening to maintain their cutting edge. This is normally performed freehand on a small oilstone of SiO_2 (Arkansas); this is a delicate and difficult procedure for an inexperienced operator. The bevel of the chisel should be laid flat on the stone with the blade forming an angle of 50–60°. The instrument is held with both hands and guided back and forth on the stone for several strokes, with emphasis on the strokes toward the edge. Sharpness may be tested by shaving the operator's fingernail. Excavators should be sharpened on their flat face by a few strokes on the stone. Sickle scalers should be sharpened on their sides to maintain adequate thickness and thus prevent bending during removal of calculus.

Alternatively, fine sandpaper discs may be used in a mandrel on a handpiece for sharpening. This is more rapid, but in inexperienced hands may lead to overtrimming of the instrument and overheating, with consequent softening of the cutting edge.

Burs should be immersed in a solution of benzalkonium chloride in an ultrasonic bath for 1 minute after use to remove adherent debris. This prolongs the cutting efficiency, particularly of diamond burs. Steel or tungsten carbide burs which have become blunt should be discarded, as should diamond burs which have been bent.

Sterilization of instruments is covered in Chapter 16 (p. 227).

5 Pulp protection

5.1 Introduction

The dental pulp is at the core of the tooth and is the tissue which formed the bulk of the tooth during its development; it continues to produce small amounts of dentine throughout life but will lay down greater amounts if stimulated by irritation. The pulp has a mass of tentacle-like projections, the odontoblast processes, which radiate into the dentinal tubules up to approximately one-third of their length. The tubules are normally patent up to the amelo-dentinal junction and are filled with tissue fluid. The pulp remains as a delicate piece of connective tissue which is easily damaged by the application of irritants to dentine.

It is therefore appropriate to regard the entire dentine as living tissue, hence the often used name dentino-pulpal complex; so it is not unexpected to find a pulpal response to irritants when they are applied to the surface of exposed dentine. It has already been shown in Chapter 1 that caries in superficial dentine produces a response in the pulp. Caries of dentine usually causes tubular sclerosis and the formation of reactionary dentine, giving the pulp some protection from subsequent operative procedures. When cavity preparation extends into dentine, anything which the operator does can damage the pulp; this is more likely where dentine unaffected by caries is encountered, i.e. at the periphery of the cavity or in some deep cavities where the pulp has not laid down defences.

All tubules lead to the pulp so the more that are involved in disease or operative treatment, the greater is the potential threat to the pulp. In the young patient, the tubules are larger and the odontoblast processes extend nearer to the amelo-dentinal junction, so the effect on the pulp is greater. Because of the protective effect of the pulpal response to caries, it is the odontoblasts under tubules at the periphery of a prepared cavity that are at greatest risk from operative procedures.

Morphologically the pulp is generally a smaller edition of the tooth, and its size normally decreases with age but will do so more in limited regions by the formation of reactionary dentine in response to caries, attrition or abrasion. Reactionary dentine is of tremendous clinical significance in the treatment of caries as it protects the pulp at the time of operative procedures and is subsequently formed in response to them. However, despite the formation of reactionary dentine, the pulp does extend closer to the surface of the tooth in certain parts; the extensions under the cusps are the pulp horns, and gingivally the pulp is closer to the surface than in the crown. In both these parts, the pulp may be encountered accidentally during cavity preparation.

5.2 Pulpitis

The pulp, being connective tissue, responds to irritants by inflammation, which may or may not resolve. Resolution is more likely with mild inflammation, while severe inflammation will usually lead to necrosis and eventually abscess formation. The condition of the pulp may be conveniently classified as:

1 Normal pulp.
2 Reversible pulpitis.
3 Irreversible pulpitis.
4 Pulpal necrosis.

This classification has a clinical basis, whereas more elaborate histopathological classifications do not correlate well with clinical findings. It should be noted that inflammatory changes in the pulp may be very localized. In an anterior tooth, part of the coronal pulp may be severely inflamed whereas the radicular pulp may be normal. In a posterior tooth, part of the coronal pulp could be necrotic while another part of the coronal pulp only several millimetres away could be mildly inflamed. These variations hinder diagnosis.

Pulpitis may be causing symptoms and is then classified as acute, or it may be symptomless and regarded as chronic; these labels do not indicate the type of inflammatory cells found in the pulp. Symptoms may range from short, sharp bouts of pain, through a continuous tolerable dull ache, to a severe throbbing pain which responds poorly to analgesics. The pain may occur through stimulation — such as eating — or be spontaneous, and its character and occurrence may change with time as reversible progresses to irreversible pulpitis, or necrosis supervenes.

Irreversible pulpitis is progressive because of the continued presence of irritants, and eventually affects the entire pulp. Inflammation will then spread beyond the pulp to involve the periapical tissues, leading to resorption of bone. If the periapical inflammation is acute, the tooth is tender and extruded from its socket, making biting on it painful. When an abscess has formed in the periapical tissues, the alveolar soft tissues over the root apices are usually swollen and the tooth may feel loose. On the other hand, chronic periapical inflammation is rarely accompanied by any symptoms.

Irritant effects on the pulp may be cumulative. Therefore, further damage by the operator to an already inflamed pulp from caries may lead to irreversible pulpitis. It is thus necessary to attempt to assess the state of the pulp before cavity preparation so that the appropriate treatment can be carried out, and the operator must be aware of the irritant effects of the various aspects of treatment.

5.3 Pulpal assessment

Prior to cavity preparation the pulp may be causing pain or, more often, it is symptomless, and in either case it is important to attain the best diagnosis of its condition. The state of the pulp is assessed from the history, clinical examination and special tests (Rowe & Pitt Ford, 1990).

The *normal pulp*, if it is a cause of pain usually through exposed dentine, is likely to produce short, sharp bouts of pain related to stimulation, such as severe change in temperature, eating, or drying of exposed dentine. Pain usually lasts a matter of a few seconds.

Reversible pulpitis, if it causes pain, is also likely to produce short, sharp bouts of pain, but of longer duration, possibly up to 1 minute, and is again caused by stimulation. There is usually a strong response to the application of cold. A common reason for the pain is exposed dentine caused by caries; by removing the carious dentine and placing a restoration, the pain is usually relieved and the pulp recovers.

Irreversible pulpitis may not cause pain, but when it does, the pain can last minutes or even hours; although it may be stimulated by eating or a change in temperature, it can occur spontaneously, during the night for example. This pain is often severe and throbbing. Because the pulp cannot recover, either the pulp or sometimes the tooth must be removed. Removal of the pulp is usually total (pulpectomy) rather than partial (pulpotomy) as the long-term result is more predictable. However, where the tooth has incompletely formed roots, pulpotomy is normally the procedure of choice to allow continued root growth.

Pulpal necrosis is not readily detectable unless it is total, but diagnosis is helped because it is often accompanied by irreversible pulpitis and there may be changes, which may be observed radiographically, in the periradicular tissues, particularly around the apex.

Where the operator is treating small carious lesions in symptomless teeth, the pulp is likely to be normal. However, where caries has caused extensive destruction of the tooth, pulpal damage must be suspected even if the pulp is not encountered during removal of carious dentine. Sometimes a heavily and apparently well-restored tooth suddenly causes pain long after placement of the restoration; the cause may be the eventual succumbing of the pulp to the original caries rather than the effect of the restorative material, recurrent caries or bacterial penetration around the restoration.

A number of clinical tests are available to assess the state of the pulp; none is absolutely reliable because the state of the pulp may vary from one part to another. Tests which may be used are:

1   Application of electric current.
2   Application of cold.
3   Application of heat.
4   Examination of radiograph.
5   Cavity preparation without anaesthesia.

APPLICATION OF ELECTRIC CURRENT

Electric current may be applied from a battery-operated 'electric pulp tester' and the intensity of current which causes a response can be recorded. It is useful to assess the level of responses from contralateral teeth. Response to a lower current than the normal contralateral tooth may indicate an inflamed pulp, whereas response solely to high current may indicate pulpal necrosis or pulpal recession. False readings can be given by leakage of current through the gingival tissues, particularly if there are metallic restorations in the tooth or the tooth is covered with saliva. Therefore, the tooth should be isolated and dried. The failure to elicit a response at the maximum output may indicate a root-filled tooth, a necrotic pulp, a receded pulp, a pulp in a state of shock following trauma, or an incomplete circuit as can occur when the operator is wearing gloves. A recent study by Bender and coworkers (1989) has shown that the lowest responses were recorded with the electrode on the incisal edge. It is very difficult to test teeth with full coverage restorations.

APPLICATION OF COLD

Cold is usually applied to a tooth by touching it intermittently with a pledget of cotton wool covered in ice crystals from evaporation of ethyl chloride; alternatively a stick of ice may be used. This often elicits a painful response in an anterior tooth because the small amount of tooth substance is cooled very rapidly; the test is less satisfactory on posterior teeth because of their greater mass. By cooling contralateral teeth, their differing responses can be assessed. A response indicates that the coronal pulp is at least partially alive or even normal. No response may mean that the coronal pulp is necrotic, the pulp has receded, insufficient cooling occurred to elicit a response in a normal pulp or the pulp is in a state of shock following recent trauma. If application of cold causes sharp pain of short duration, it indicates a normal or reversibly inflamed pulp. If it causes a prolonged burst of agonizing pain, it indicates irreversible pulpitis.

APPLICATION OF HEAT

Heat is usually applied by a heated stick of gutta-percha being dabbed intermittently onto the tooth surface previously smeared with vaseline. A response indicates that some part of the pulp is alive. Heat has been regarded as being particularly effective in diagnosing a pulp with irreversible pulpitis when it has failed to respond to the application of cold; however, this was not supported in a clinical study by Dummer *et al.* (1980). Lack of response may occur for similar reasons as lack of response to cold.

EXAMINATION OF RADIOGRAPHS

Examination of a good quality bitewing radiograph provides useful indicators of the pulpal condition by showing two-dimensionally the extent of caries, the presence of recurrent caries, the amount of reactionary dentine, the size of the pulp chamber and evidence of internal resorption. A periapical radiograph provides additional information about periradicular radiolucencies. In teeth with large cavities, the distance between the base of the cavity and the pulp is small and irritants can therefore readily affect the pulp. The formation of reactionary dentine in response to caries indicates that the pulp may have responded successfully to the carious attack; however, an abnormally large shadow of the pulp on a radiograph suggests that pulpal necrosis occurred at an earlier age. A periapical radiolucency indicates that most, if not all, of the pulp is necrotic, for which removal of the pulp would be required.

CAVITY PREPARATION

Cavity preparation without anaesthesia may give an indication of the state of the pulp. It is only used when all the other tests have failed to give a diagnosis. Cavity preparation may even fail to elicit a painful response in a tooth with a vital pulp if the tubules being drilled do not connect with odontoblast processes, as a result of tubular sclerosis or deposition of reactionary dentine.

DIAGNOSIS

Having carried out all these tests the clinician hopes that he can arrive at a diagnosis, but he cannot always be certain that it is correct. Where the diagnosis is uncertain in a symptomless tooth, it is usual to assume that the pulp is normal in the absence of definite contrary evidence. However, in a tooth which previously caused symptoms, and on which it is planned to place a crown, it would be most appropriate to assume that the pulp has been irreversibly damaged and carry out root treatment. Where the operator cannot decide which of several teeth is causing pain, a wait and see policy is appropriate to prevent unnecessary treatment to the wrong tooth.

5.4 Pulpal irritants

These may be considered in the following groups:
1   Original condition.
2   Cavity preparation.
3   Materials.
4   Bacterial leakage.
The harmful effects of these are considered to be cumulative; therefore, they should be minimized as far as possible.

ORIGINAL CONDITION

Caries is a major pulpal irritant and has been covered in Chapter 1. Attrition, abrasion and erosion are less common causes of pulpal irritation and have been considered in Chapter 3; they frequently cause the formation of reactionary dentine and tubular sclerosis. The dentine exposed by wear is usually insensitive and irritants applied to it rarely affect the pulp. Dentine exposed by traumatic injury is quite different, for the tubules are patent and irritants applied to the dentine surface can readily cause a severe pulpal reaction; the exposed dentine is also painful to touch. The exposed surface can rapidly become covered by bacterial plaque, the micro-organisms of which and their toxins can penetrate the dentinal tubules, resulting in irreversible pulpitis; traumatic injuries have been covered in Chapter 3.

CAVITY PREPARATION

The preparation of teeth for restorations using rotary instruments can have a very harmful effect on the pulp unless precautionary measures are taken. It has even been stated that 'decay in many instances is much less harmful than the operative procedure used to treat it' (Seltzer & Bender, 1984).

A number of studies have clearly shown that pulpal damage is far greater when the dentine is drilled dry than with waterspray, especially at high bur speeds. Pulpal damage can also occur when a considerable thickness of dentine remains between the cavity and the pulp. This may be explained by the mechanism of the pulpal response. The tubules are fine capillary channels containing, for the most part, tissue fluid. During cavity preparation without coolant, heat is generated by the bur, causing evaporation of water from the open ends of affected tubules. Capillary action draws fluid out of the pulp into the tubules. If evaporation is rapid, odontoblasts become sucked into the tubules and mechano-receptor nerve fibres become stretched, causing pain. Excess heat may lead to extensive aspiration of odontoblasts into tubules and they may subsequently undergo necrosis.

The harmful effect of rotary instruments becomes pronounced as more heat is generated. For this reason it is essential to use waterspray at all but the very slowest speeds. The turbine handpiece should never be used without waterspray. The use of airspray alone is an unacceptable alternative, as the air blast desiccates the dentine causing pulpal damage and is not such an effective coolant.

When using waterspray, it is essential to ensure that the spray is directed in sufficient volume at the dentine being cut. The pulp is particularly vulnerable during the starting and stopping of the turbine, for at these times the waterspray is likely to be insufficient. If the operator smells burning during tooth preparation, there is inadequate coolant and pulpal damage will inevitably follow.

The greater the surface area of dentine involved, the more likely is pulpal damage. Therefore, with large cavities and particularly with extracoronal preparations, the pulp is at great risk.

As the cavity gets deeper into dentine, the tubules are closer together and of wider diameter so pulpal effects can be more pronounced. Close to the pulp, the bur will cut odontoblast processes, causing further tissue damage.

Heat from a bur will cause a far greater effect on the pulp by capillary action than by conduction, because dentine is a good insulator and the small amount of heat generated is rapidly dissipated.

Cavities can be taken close to the pulp without permanent damage using burs at any speed provided that waterspray cooling is effective, the subsequent filling material is non-irritant and there is no bacterial contamination at the time of preparation or, more importantly, afterwards.

The use of a short blast of compressed air from a 3-in-1 syringe to dry a cavity appears to be acceptable. However, prolonged drying by excessive use of the air syringe or by leaving the isolated tooth to dry out will cause aspiration of odontoblasts into the tubules. This is undesirable and should be avoided.

MATERIALS

There is a great volume of literature on the harmful effects on the pulp of a number of dental materials. Brännström (1982) has suggested that the unfavourable pulpal response may, in many instances, be due to the clinical usage of the materials rather than the materials themselves being irritant.

There is general agreement that amalgam, gold and porcelain are non-irritant. Resin-based materials (unfilled and composite resins), glass ionomer cement, zinc phosphate cement and silicate cement have been widely regarded as irritant in varying degrees to the pulp, but Cox and co-workers (1987) have shown that most of the pulpal responses to these materials occur because of bacterial penetration between the restoration and the cavity wall and that responses are rarely due to chemical irritation.

BACTERIAL LEAKAGE

Many plastic restorations are either not bonded at all to the tooth or if there is bonding it does not occur around the entire cavity margin and, as a result of shrinkage on setting and a different coefficient of thermal expansion from enamel, a microspace often exists between the restoration and tooth. This can become colonized by bacteria, which may grow into the dentinal tubules or bacterial toxins may diffuse down the tubules to cause pulpal inflammation. The effect on the pulp will depend on the number of patent dentinal tubules, the extent of bacterial penetration, the types of bacteria and the existing condition of the pulp. The pulp may be able to respond by tubular sclerosis and formation of reactionary dentine so that after some weeks the bacteria cease to cause irritation. However, a number of measures should be taken to reduce the harmful pulpal effects from these bacteria while the pulp is most vulnerable. A lining may be placed over the open tubules to block their ends, and the cavity walls may be coated with a resinous material to seal the interface, or the restorative material may be bonded to the tooth, or an adhesive material may be used to restore the tooth.

It is important that exposed dentinal tubules in a preparation for a rigid restoration should be protected by a temporary restoration which seals effectively during the interval between preparation and insertion of the rigid restoration. Failure to do so may lead to irreversible pulpitis.

5.5 Linings

FUNCTION OF LINING

The most important function of a lining is to protect the pulp under a restoration; subsidiary functions are structural, therapeutic and adhesive. In North America, the term *base* is used instead of *lining*, and *cavity liner* describes a suspension of calcium hydroxide or zinc oxide in a varnish.

The major protective role of a lining is to prevent the bacteria usually present around a restoration or their toxins from entering the tubules and irritating the pulp. The lining is applied as a thin layer to cover the exposed tubules on pulpal, axial and gingival walls; this latter wall is particularly important as the number of tubules per square millimetre is very high and there may be little reactionary dentine under these tubules. It is very beneficial if the lining material is bacteriostatic.

Another role is to protect the pulp from irritant restorative materials, so it is essential that the lining material itself is non-irritant.

Metallic restorations are conductors of heat and for many years it has been considered desirable to place a lining to insulate the pulp from thermal shock. Braden in 1964 doubted the benefit of such a procedure, as he found that dentine was a better insulator than available lining materials which were only effective in thick sections; most linings under restorations are thin in cross-section. Brännström (1986) has supported the view, which is contrary to traditional teaching, that a lining even in a deep cavity is unnecessary to protect the pulp from thermal shock. Most thermal changes are of short duration as the small amount of heat in hot food is rapidly dissipated to the surrounding tissues.

Linings have long been regarded as having a valuable structural function. This aspect has often been overstated, as most linings do not improve the resistance form of the cavity because they have little or no adhesion to the underlying dentine. In Fig. 5.1, the restoration and lining should be regarded as functioning as one unit. It has been suggested that an uneven pulpal floor of an occlusal cavity should be levelled with lining material to improve cavity form, but it is of no clinical benefit. Structural linings have been proposed to reduce the bulk of expensive restorative material, but invariably the small saving of material is not recouped in the extra time taken to mix, place and shape the lining material. The structural use of linings is to eliminate undercuts from preparations for rigid restorations and this reduces the amount of sound tooth substance which otherwise would need to be removed to establish a preparation of correct taper.

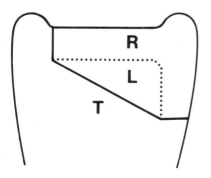

Fig. 5.1 The lining will not improve the resistance form of the cavity for the restoration, because it is unlikely to have good adhesion to the underlying dentine.

The adhesive function of a lining is more a desire than clinical reality, as, apart from glass ionomer cement, no lining material bonds to dentine. A durable bond will require conditioning of the dentine surface to remove the smear layer. The concept is not new as it was proposed by Baldwin in 1897. He packed amalgam onto a partially set lining to obtain mechanical interlocking. The technique is difficult to do well and can easily result in cement being displaced to the margins, where it may subsequently dissolve, creating a site for recurrent caries or corrosion of the amalgam.

Linings have an indirect therapeutic role by controlling caries and allowing reparative processes in the pulp to occur. This role will be considered under treatment of deep caries and pulpal exposures.

CHOICE OF LINING MATERIAL

Calcium hydroxide cements have been the most widely used lining materials in recent years as they combine several properties — an initial antibacterial effect, non-irritancy even when applied directly to the pulp, and adequate strength. They are usually presented as two pastes; one contains calcium hydroxide in an inert liquid while the other contains a salicylate. When similar amounts of each paste are mixed, a cement of calcium salicylate is formed. The freshly mixed cement has a creamy consistency and can be applied easily to the dentine surfaces of a cavity with a small ball-ended instrument. It sets rapidly and, because of its relatively low strength, any excess may be trimmed away with a sharp excavator after setting. The cement is compatible with available restorative materials, although it is best not used as the sole lining material under elastomeric impressions for rigid restorations, because it may be pulled away from the dentine during removal of the impression from the teeth. Provided that the lining is not exposed to saliva or plaque, it will not dissolve; however, should part of the tooth or restoration fail, causing exposure of the cement to saliva and plaque, it can rapidly dissolve and in certain circumstances may allow spread of caries under such a restoration and even lead to pulpal involvement.

Cements based on zinc oxide–eugenol may also be used as lining materials. The cements are almost always used in a modified form to increase the speed of set and achieve sufficient strength; they are usually presented as a powder consisting mainly of zinc oxide; and a liquid which is principally eugenol. Sufficient powder is mixed with a drop of liquid (approximate powder : liquid ratio, 4 : 1) to give a putty consistency. At this consistency it may be applied to most cavities, causing little or no pulpal response. This favourable response is mainly due to the cement's bacteriostatic properties and its ability to prevent bacterial penetration around it, although eugenol itself is mildly irritant. A small piece of the mixed cement is conveyed to the cavity on the tip of a probe and tamped into place with a burnisher or plugger. Any excess material should be removed with an excavator before it has set, or after setting with a bur in a low-speed handpiece. The eugenol in the recently inserted lining interferes with the setting of resin-based restorative materials so zinc oxide–eugenol cement should not be used directly under these materials. Because the cement has good sealing ability and antibacterial effects, it is widely used as an effective temporary filling material.

Zinc phosphate cement has been extensively used as a lining material for many years. However, a number of studies have indicated that it can irritate the pulp, although the exact cause has been unclear (Plant & Jones, 1976). There is increasing evidence to indicate that the cement's setting shrinkage allows bacteria to leak around the lining; and this is now considered to be the principal cause of its pulpal irritation in experimental studies (Watts, 1979). Glass ionomer cement has also been advocated as a lining cement on the grounds of adhesion. To obtain the maximum effect, the dentine must first be conditioned to remove the smear layer. It is compatible with resin-based restorative materials; however, it is not antibacterial.

Copal resin varnish is a solution of a natural resin in an organic solvent such as acetone, chloroform or ether. It is normally applied to the walls of a cavity prepared for amalgam to reduce the leakage of fluids and bacteria along the interface of restoration and cavity wall. It is usually placed on the cavity walls by a pledget of cotton wool held in tweezers. A minimum of two coats is required to compensate for the gaps produced in the varnish film as the solvent evaporates. Unlike lining cements, it is acceptable and normal practice to allow copalite varnish to extend to the cavity margins. The varnish is effective in reducing leakage around a newly inserted amalgam restoration. It should be noted that after some months, leakage around amalgam restorations in unvarnished cavities becomes reduced as a result of corrosion. The use of varnish in cavities for composite resin restorations is not advised as the solvent may interfere with setting of the restorative material. Varnish would also reduce the effectiveness of etching solutions on cavity margins in the acid-etch technique. If the varnish thickens in its bottle on storage, it may be diluted with more solvent.

Cavity varnishes have been proposed as the sole method of pulpal protection from restorations and associated bacterial leakage; they have been shown to be effective under certain clinical conditions: the cavity surface needs to be thoroughly clean and dry and coated with a special varnish which gives a thick film (Nordenvall *et al.*, 1979). The general view is that a lining cement together with the use of copalite varnish is preferable to copalite varnish alone, as they are likely to be more effective.

It has been shown that application of phosphoric acid to cavities in the acid-etch technique does not in itself cause pulpal irritation but the subsequent bacterial leakage which could occur around the restoration does. If the acid contacts dentine, it widens the orifices of tubules, allowing easier bacterial penetration toward the pulp. With many clinical cavities there may be no cervical wall of enamel into which the composite resin can bond, thus the peripheral seal is incomplete and a potential route exists for bacteria to enter the cavity wall microspace. It is therefore advisable to cover the dentine with a calcium hydroxide cement before application of the etching acid to prevent the orifices of the tubules being opened. After applying the acid, it may be necessary to reapply lining cement where it has been removed by the acid.

5.6 Treatment of deep caries and pulpal exposures

There is general agreement that all carious dentine should be removed from the amelo-dentinal junction at the cavity margin; however, there has been less agreement over whether all the carious dentine overlying the pulp should be removed. In a tooth which is considered to have a healthy pulp, the prognosis for the pulp is better if accidental exposure during removal of carious dentine is avoided.

There is clinical evidence to support the leaving of a small amount of carious dentine over the pulp under a well-executed restoration as the caries becomes arrested (Fairbourn *et al.*, 1980). However, as restorations do not seal, some people regard leaving carious dentine as a dangerous procedure inviting further spread of the lesion. Shovelton (1968) showed that only 64% of clinically hard dentine floors were bacteria-free, while 28% of soft dentine floors were bacteria-free. Therefore, in a third of teeth where the clinician thought he had a clean floor, he was wrong, and in a quarter of teeth where he thought he needed to remove more softened dentine, bacteria were absent. Fusayama (1979) offered a rational solution to this problem by using a caries indicator dye (e.g. 1% Acid Red in propanol) in the prepared cavity. The dye stains the infected dentine bright red but leaves the deeper demineralized dentine unstained. The unstained demineralized dentine has the capacity to remineralize, thereby justifying its retention. After removal of the stained dentine, an antibacterial lining (e.g. zinc oxide–eugenol cement) should be placed as it slowly leaches eugenol which will kill any remaining bacteria; calcium hydroxide cements are not so effective. If caries has spread to the pulp, then at least the superficial part of the pulp is likely to be necrotic and irreversibly damaged. Often, such a tooth may have had a history of prolonged pain, or on removal of caries, the pulp chamber is uncovered, surrounded by carious dentine; this is termed a carious exposure. The exposed pulp chamber may be empty, contain pus or bleed profusely. The pulp cannot be kept alive and root canal treatment is normally required to retain the tooth.

The pulp may be exposed traumatically during incorrect cavity preparation. In this situation, the pulp has a good chance of remaining vital provided that the bur did not enter the pulp and mutilate it and provided that the wound did not become contaminated by saliva, plaque or carious dentine at the time of injury or subsequently. By placing a calcium hydroxide cement material over the exposed intact pulp, a reactionary dentine barrier is likely to form within a few months; most studies have shown at least a 75% success rate. For long-term success it is essential to place a zinc oxide–eugenol cement lining over the calcium hydroxide cement (Langer *et al.*, 1970), otherwise success is jeopardized (Cox *et al.*, 1985). The use of zinc oxide–eugenol cement for direct placement on the exposed pulp is not nearly so successful, because eugenol is irritant when applied directly to tissue.

Bibliography

Bender I. B., Landau M. A., Fonsecca S. & Trowbridge H. O. (1989) The optimum placement-site of the electrode in electric pulp testing of the 12 anterior teeth. *Journal of the American Dental Association*, **118**, 305–310.

Braden M. (1964) Heat conduction in teeth and the effect of lining materials. *Journal of Dental Research*, **43**, 315–322.

Brännström M. (1982) *Dentin and Pulp in Restorative Dentistry*. Wolfe Medical Publications, London.

Brännström M. (1986) The cause of post restorative sensitivity and its prevention. *Journal of Endodontics*, **12**, 475–481.

Brännström M. & Nordenvall K. J. (1978) Bacterial penetration, pulpal reaction and the inner surface of Concise Enamel Bond. Composite fillings in etched and unetched cavities. *Journal of Dental Research*, **57**, 3–10.

Cox C. F., Bergenholtz G., Heyes D. R., Syed S. A., Fitzgerald M. & Heys R. J. (1985) Pulp capping of the dental pulp mechanically exposed to the oral microflora. A 1–2 year observation of wound healing in the monkey. *Journal of Oral Pathology*, **14**, 156–168.

Cox C. F., Keall C. L., Keall H. J., Ostro E. & Bergenholtz G. (1987) Biocompatibility of surface-sealed dental materials against exposed pulps. *Journal of Prosthetic Dentistry*, **57**, 1–8.

Dummer P. M. H., Hicks R. & Huws D. (1980) Clinical signs and symptoms in pulp disease. *International Endodontic Journal*, **13**, 27–35.

Fairbourn D. R., Charbeneau G. T. & Loesche W. J. (1980) Effect of Improved Dycal and IRM on bacteria in deep carious lesions. *Journal of the American Dental Association*, **100**, 547–552.

Fusayama T. (1979) Two layers of carious dentin: diagnosis and treatment. *Operative Dentistry*, **4**, 63–70.

Langer M., Ulmansky M. & Sela J. (1970) Behaviour of human dental pulp to Calxyl with or without zinc oxide eugenol. *Archives of Oral Biology*, **15**, 189–194.

Nordenvall K. J., Brännström M. & Torstensson B. (1979) Pulp reactions and micro-organisms under ASPA and Concise Composite fillings. *Journal of Dentistry for Children*, **46**, 449–453.

Paterson R. C. & Watts A. (1981) Caries, bacteria, the pulp and plastic restorations. *British Dental Journal*, **151**, 54–58.

Plant C. G. & Jones D. W. (1976) The damaging effects of restorative materials. Part 2. Pulpal effects related to physical and chemical properties. *British Dental Journal*, **140**, 406–412.

Rowe A. H. R. & Pitt Ford T. R. (1990) The assessment of pulpal vitality. *International Endodontic Journal*, **23**, 77–83.

Seltzer S. & Bender I. B. (1984) *The Dental Pulp. Biologic Considerations in Dental Procedures*, 3rd edn. Lippincott, Philadelphia.

Shovelton D. S. (1968) A study of deep carious dentine. *International Dental Journal*, **18**, 392–405.

Watts A. (1979) Bacterial contamination and the toxicity of silicate and zinc phosphate cements. *British Dental Journal*, **146**, 7–13.

6 Principles of treating dental caries

6.1 Introduction

In the first chapter the aetiology and pathology of dental caries were considered, followed by the prevention and control of the disease in the second chapter. When the disease has progressed beyond the stage of just being controlled, treatment is required to remove the affected enamel and dentine and to restore the defect in the tooth, so returning it to function. The surgical treatment and insertion of a restoration can only be successful in the long term if the environment in the mouth is suitable, i.e. there is reform of diet and control of plaque.

Before commencing treatment the patient should have a positive attitude to dental care and treatment, because treatment is more successful in a patient who has a low incidence of caries and is a regular attender. However, some regular attenders present with a high incidence of caries, and to achieve dental health dietary analysis and advice is essential. For patients who have a low prevalence of caries in their mouths, cavities that need to be prepared can often be very conservative because the likelihood of further caries is low.

The whole mouth must be examined and an overall plan of treatment evolved before individual teeth are restored (Chapter 16). If there is pulpal, periapical or periodontal disease then these should be treated or at least controlled prior to permanent restoration of the teeth. Where periodontal disease has been severe, then the affected teeth might need to be extracted whatever the extent of dental caries in them. However, where the periodontal condition is less severe, caries in a tooth should be removed and a temporary restoration placed until the periodontal disease is controlled or treated. Where a non-functional tooth, such as an over-erupted upper third molar, is affected by caries there is no purpose in restoring it; indeed, the distal surface of the second molar becomes more readily cleansable by its removal. Furthermore, for the operator, removal of the tooth is considerably easier than restoring it.

In a child it may be better to extract a grossly carious first permanent molar rather than a sound premolar if one tooth in the quadrant must be extracted to alleviate crowding as part of orthodontic treatment.

Once the surface of a carious lesion in enamel has collapsed to form a cavity and the dentine has become invaded by bacteria, the use of preventive measures alone is unlikely to arrest spread of the lesion in dentine. The decayed part of the tooth should then be removed and replaced by a suitable restorative material. Because spread of caries is usually more extensive in dentine than in enamel, removal of decay produces a *cavity* and so a *filling* or *intracoronal restoration* is the most appropriate way of restoring the tooth. Where decay is extensive, the remaining cusps may be weakened such that some form of extracoronal restoration is required to prevent the tooth from being split apart.

The operator may not always examine the patient's tooth until a considerable amount of dentine has been destroyed by caries. In some instances caries may be so extensive that restoration of the tooth is impractical and extraction is the only treatment.

The bulk of the tooth is composed of dentine, a tough elastic material, which absorbs the forces exerted on teeth during the chewing of food and during tooth contact. Dentine is a soft material which would wear rapidly if it were exposed on the occlusal surface. However, by being covered, or veneered, with a layer of extremely hard but brittle enamel, tooth wear is normally reduced to an insignificant amount. The enamel also protects the dentine from bacterial invasion and the pulp from the consequences of that. If the whole tooth were composed of enamel, it would be too brittle and would crack under masticatory forces. Whenever a cavity is prepared in the occlusal surface of a tooth, it is weakened; and the larger the cavity, the weaker is the remaining tooth. Therefore, all cavities should be kept as small as possible with minimal loss of sound tooth substance.

The purpose of cavity preparation is to remove the decayed enamel and dentine, and secondly to shape the tooth to retain the restoration. Retention of materials is achieved in different ways; one large group of materials, which includes amalgam, is wedged physically in the cavity because the dimensions of the cavity within the tooth are greater than those at the surface. A second group, comprising adhesive materials, is retained by the material's adhesion to mineralized dental tissue and therefore requires a large enough surface to which to bond. A third group, which includes cast gold, being solid at the time of placement, requires a preparation of the tooth which is tapered to allow insertion of the restoration and which resists displacement of the restoration; the restoration is kept in place by a cement lute.

Enamel at the periphery of a carious lesion is often unsupported by sound dentine, because caries tends to spread out along the amelo-dentinal junction. In general, this unsupported enamel should be removed during cavity preparation to prevent its fracture from applied forces after a restoration has been placed. Pressure may be applied to unsupported enamel directly by opposing teeth in occlusal contacts, indirectly through the restoration, by thermal expansion of a metallic restoration or setting contraction of a resin-based material. Because drilling of sound dentine may injure the pulp, only a minimal amount of sound dentine should be removed during cavity preparation.

6.2 Stages of cavity preparation

The preparation of a cavity should always be carried out in an orderly manner, and the stages were originally described by Black early this century. It is notable how little these stages have changed over the years, although emphasis on certain aspects has altered. Fundamentally the principles were correct and they hold good for all sizes of lesions. At the turn of the century many patients had large untreated carious lesions, whereas now in Britain dental caries tends to be detected and treated much earlier. Also, the aetiology and prevention of caries have become better understood.

Black was concerned with preventing the recurrence of caries around restorations so he deliberately overenlarged cavities, particularly those involving caries on smooth surfaces, to include high risk areas. Over the years the recommended size of these cavities has decreased, since extension of cavities did not result in prevention, smaller cavities weaken teeth less and much greater emphasis is now placed on dietary advice and plaque control. The size is now determined by the extent of caries present.

The stages are:
1 Access.
2 Removal of superficial caries.
3 Resistance form.
4 Retention.
5 Convenience form.
6 Margins.
7 Removal of deep caries.
8 Cavity toilet.

ACCESS

There are three aspects to this: first, allowing the operator to see the extent of the caries; secondly, allowing the bur to reach the carious dentine at the amelo-dentinal junction; and thirdly, allowing the waterspray to reach the tip of the bur.

The first stage of cavity preparation is to gain access to the carious lesion in dentine. Where caries has affected, for example, the buccal surface of the tooth, then loss of enamel may have achieved this without the need to use dental instruments. However, where caries has affected the enamel on the approximal surface, direct access is normally prevented by the presence of the adjacent tooth. Therefore, it is necessary to drill through sound enamel on the inner aspect of the marginal ridge to reach the carious dentine. In the early dentine approximal lesion, it is possible to preserve intact the marginal ridge supported by sound dentine. In the larger lesion the carious process has often removed dentinal support from the enamel marginal ridge, so this enamel would need to be removed anyway.

REMOVAL OF SUPERFICIAL CARIES

The extent of the cavity at the surface of the tooth is mainly governed by the extent of caries. When enamel is completely carious, it is absent, while partially carious enamel has an opaque chalky colour and is friable; carious enamel must be removed and none is permitted to remain at the cavity margin with the possible exception of lesions on the buccal surface in a highly motivated patient. Carious dentine is usually a darker colour and always noticeably softer than sound dentine and it must be removed from the amelo-dentinal junction. The operator will find it helpful to stain the residual carious dentine with a dye, e.g. 1% Acid Red in propanol. Two groups of workers have found that the use of dye disclosed caries which otherwise would have been missed. Because of the lateral spread of caries at the amelo-dentinal junction, it is usual for carious dentine to be overlaid by sound enamel, which with few exceptions must be removed as it is unsupported. Therefore, it is the extent of caries in *dentine* which determines cavity size. The removal of enamel increases the size of the cavity but by limiting removal to unsupported prisms, unnecessary overextension is prevented (Fig. 6.1).

Where a cavity involves a fissure system of a tooth, most frequently because of caries in some part, it has been usual practice to extend the cavity along the fissure to include the rest of the system for the following reasons: first, bacterial penetration may be present at the amelo-dentinal junction but undetected; second, it is extremely difficult to finish the margins of a restoration in a deep fissure; third, such a fissure is at high risk of subsequent caries; and finally, it is considerably easier to extend the cavity by a small amount along the fissure at the time of initial preparation rather than find it necessary to replace the restoration within a year or two. This extension into fissures which are not deemed carious is given the name 'extension for prevention'. As with so many aspects of dentistry, it is a two-edged sword; it can work to the benefit of the patient or, if done injudiciously, can lead to unnecessary destruction of tooth substance with significant

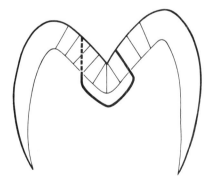

Fig. 6.1 The removal of enamel affects cavity size. On the right hand side the cavity wall is based on prism angulation, while on the left hand side the dotted cavity wall would unnecessarily remove enamel.

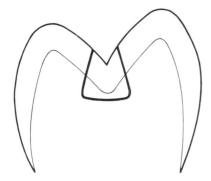

Fig. 6.2 The cavity floor is placed just within dentine in the same plane as the occlusal surface to provide resistance to displacement. The cavity walls converge occlusally to provide retention.

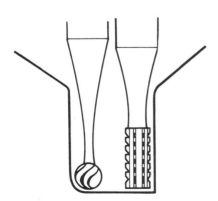

Fig. 6.3 A small round bur creates a rounded line angle whereas a fissure bur creates a sharp line angle.

weakening of cusps and enamel ridges, particularly the marginal ridges. Where extension for prevention is carried out, the width of these extensions up cusp slopes in sound fissures should be as small as possible and is governed by the *smallest* size of bur available.

In the last decade, the 'Preventive Resin Restoration' has been proposed to deal with early fissure caries. Only carious enamel (and dentine) is removed, and a fissure sealant is placed over the composite resin restoration and remaining sound fissures (page 91).

Where cavities involve the smooth surfaces of teeth, the extension of these cavities into cleansable or 'safe' areas was proposed in the past; such overextension is now regarded as unacceptable because plaque may happily grow on enamel in these 'cleansable' areas as well as interproximally. The subgingival extension of a cavity was considered to place the margin in an area safe from caries, but once the junctional epithelium has become detached from enamel it will not reattach to the restoration. The margin of the restoration is never as smooth as sound enamel and accumulates more plaque, so the cavity should not be extended subgingivally unless the presence of caries dictates.

RESISTANCE FORM

All restorations are subject to displacing forces, those on the occlusal surface being the most severe. Therefore, the cavity must be shaped to prevent the restoration being bitten out or displaced by vigorous brushing. For a cavity confined to the occlusal surface of a tooth this is usually achieved by preparing a pulpal floor just within dentine in the same plane as the occlusal surface. The opposing side walls of the cavity should be angled to the floor, although the corners, or line angles, do not need to be sharp (Fig. 6.2). Sharp line angles are considered to induce stress in the remaining tooth, therefore slightly rounded line angles are better; these may be created by a small round (or pear-shaped) bur (Fig. 6.3). Use of a *large* round bur would create poor resistance form and must be avoided. Where the cavity additionally involves the approximal surface, the gingival wall is usually prepared perpendicular to the long axis of the tooth (Fig. 6.4) or it may slope inwards. If the gingival wall were to slope towards the cavity margin, then forces applied to the marginal ridge would tend to cause the proximal part of the restoration to move out and fracture from the occlusal part. Besides vertical displacement, such restorations may be displaced proximally unless the cavity is shaped to prevent this. A dovetail is often created by following the natural contour of the fissure system (Fig. 6.5), or retentive grooves are placed in the dentine walls of

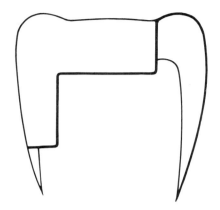

Fig. 6.4 The gingival and pulpal (occlusal) walls should be prepared perpendicular to the long axis of the tooth to resist displacement.

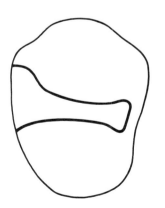

Fig. 6.5 By following the fissure system a dovetail may be placed away from the proximal part.

the proximal part; this latter is only possible when a small lesion is being treated and is also difficult to accomplish.

RETENTION

This may be considered as resistance to removal along the line of insertion. For the majority of plastic restorations the cavity is made larger internally than at the surface, and is achieved by angling the walls of the cavity so that they converge occlusally, i.e. undercut (Fig. 6.2). The cavity is normally widest at the amelo-dentinal junction or just within the dentine; widening the cavity at a deeper level could result in unnecessary pulpal damage or even exposure.

Where the cavity must be tapered to allow insertion of a rigid restoration, e.g. in cast gold, retention is increased if the angle of taper is small, the walls are long and the wall area of the preparation is as large as possible. Further retention may be gained by placing tapered grooves in the walls.

CONVENIENCE FORM

The enlargement of a cavity for ease of the operator is now considered unacceptable. However, where sound enamel must be removed because it overlies carious dentine, then its early removal will create improved access to the caries, allowing the operator to see and place his instruments more accurately. In small cavities, instruments should be chosen to fit the cavity rather than the cavity needing to be widened to accommodate large instruments.

MARGINS

By this stage no carious enamel should remain and the dentine at the periphery of the cavity should be free from caries. For restorations with amalgam, a simple butt joint at the cavity margin is required because amalgam is brittle. The enamel at the cavity margin must be trimmed to remove unsupported prisms, otherwise they would fracture either during placement of the restoration or shortly afterwards. However, for cast gold restorations, the margin of the restoration is finished as a thin edge to allow the malleable metal to be adapted after casting; this requires a bevel to be prepared along the enamel margin where possible.

REMOVAL OF DEEP CARIES

The only place where caries should now be present is on the walls or floor of the cavity closest to the pulp, and the carious dentine should be carefully removed in layers with a medium-sized round bur (ISO size 012) in a low-speed handpiece or with a hand excavator. Carious dentine should readily come away because it is softer than sound dentine. Where the caries has not penetrated deeply, the translucent mineralized zone should provide a hard convenient limit to the extent of cavity preparation; however, with more extensive caries such a barrier is likely to have been demineralized. It has long been argued whether or not it is permissible to leave carious dentine in a cavity under a restoration in a symptomless tooth without signs of irreversible pulpitis. Certainly caries does occasionally remain under well-executed restorations without causing undesirable sequelae. However, the amount left is small and the lesion is remote from the margins and covered by a stable lining and well-fitting restoration. Success may occur because the deepest softened layer of the lesion is sterile, or if infected dentine was left the cariogenic bacteria are effectively sealed from nutrients, or the lining material may have had a bacteriostatic effect. Removal of the entire carious lesion could have resulted in pulpal exposure, following which continued vitality of the pulp would have been uncertain. In clinical practice, the operator should apply a caries indicator dye and remove the brightly stained dentine which is infected. Any soft but colourless remaining dentine should be left as it is not infected. This approach should avoid unnecessary pulpal exposure and is far less empirical than judging when to stop. However, when the patient has experienced irreversible pulpitis, all the carious dentine should be removed right into the pulp as a prelude to root canal treatment.

In deep cavities, particularly under old restorations, the base of the cavity may be composed of reactionary dentine, which is considerably darker than normal dentine and similar in colour to carious dentine but is substantially harder; it should not be removed, as it is unnecessary and the pulp could be close underneath.

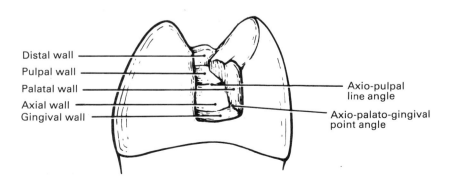

Distal wall
Pulpal wall
Palatal wall
Axial wall
Gingival wall

Axio-pulpal line angle
Axio-palato-gingival point angle

Fig. 6.6 The walls of the cavity are given specific names; line angles are derived from adjacent surfaces as are point angles.

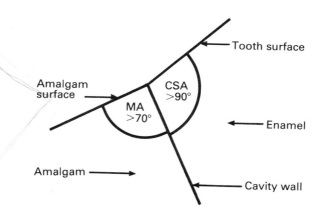

Fig. 6.7 The cavo-surface angle (CSA) must not be less than 90°; for amalgam the margin angle (MA) should not be less than 70°.

CAVITY TOILET

The preparation of the cavity should now be complete. Any debris in the cavity is washed away with the waterspray prior to drying the cavity with the airspray. The cavity should be carefully examined from different aspects for defects; any errors which are found must be corrected. The tooth is then ready for restoration. In the past, various medicaments were recommended for swabbing the cavity, but the current consensus is that many are likely to be more irritant than beneficial, or to provide short-lived benefit.

6.3 Cavity nomenclature

The reader should refer to Fig. 6.6. The surfaces of cavities are called walls or floors, and two of particular note are the pulpal floor (or wall) and the axial wall. This nomenclature was developed by Black.

Where two walls meet, a line angle is formed and its name is derived from the adjacent surfaces; common examples are the axio-pulpal line angle and the cavo-surface angle. The cavo-surface angle occurs where any cavity wall meets the surface of the tooth, although in most descriptions the important point is its size at a particular place. For amalgam restorations the cavo-surface angle must not be less than 90°, and is frequently over 110° on the occlusal surface (Fig. 6.7). It is often considered in conjunction with the margin angle of the restoration; this is the angle that the surface of the restoration makes with the cavity wall. The margin angle for amalgam on the occlusal surface should not be less than 70° otherwise the fine amalgam margin will chip (Elderton, 1984). The sum of cavo-surface and margin angles may not always be 180°. Where three walls meet, a point angle is formed and its name is derived from the three adjacent surfaces; this term is not widely used. An example is shown in Fig. 6.6.

Bibliography

Black G. V. (1917) *A Work on Operative Dentistry*, 3rd edn, Vol. 2. Medico-Dental Publishing Co., Chicago.

Elderton R. J. (1984) New approaches to cavity design. *British Dental Journal*, **157**, 421–427.

Elderton R. J. (1984) Cavo-surface angles, amalgam margin angles and occlusal cavity preparations. *British Dental Journal*, **156**, 319–324.

Kidd E. A. M., Joyston-Bechal S., Smith M. M., Allan R., Howe L. C. & Smith S. R. (1989) The use of a caries detector dye in cavity preparation. *British Dental Journal*, **167**, 132–134.

7 Properties of plastic restorative materials

7.1 Introduction

The aim of restorative treatment is not only to remove the diseased tooth substance and prevent the recurrence of caries but also to restore the tooth to function. The ideal restorative material does not exist but the reader should be familiar with the most desirable properties so that comparison can be made with those of materials which are in use, and new materials which will become available.

Two properties which are fundamental are that the material should be easy to use and it should be long lasting. In addition the material should:

1 have adequate strength, both compressive and tensile;
2 be insoluble and non-corrodible in the mouth;
3 have a low exotherm and negligible change of volume on setting;
4 be non-toxic and non-irritant to pulpal and gingival tissues;
5 be trimmed and polished without difficulty;
6 have a rate of wear similar to that of enamel;
7 have an ability to protect adjacent tooth substance from a recurrence of caries;
8 have a coefficient of thermal expansion similar to that of enamel and dentine;
9 have a thermal diffusivity similar to that of enamel and dentine;
10 have a low water absorption;
11 be adhesive to tooth substance;
12 be radiopaque;
13 have a similar colour and translucency to tooth substance;
14 have a good shelf-life;
15 be inexpensive.

The available restorative materials may be placed into two groups, *rigid* and *plastic*, depending on their state at the time of placement.

The rigid restorative materials, of which cast gold is an example, are formed into a restoration outside the mouth and this is placed in a rigid state into or onto the prepared tooth. These materials are extensively used for extracoronal restorations which are retained by the shape of the preparation and assisted by a cement lute; they will be considered in detail in Chapter 10.

The plastic restorative materials are placed into prepared cavities in teeth while they are soft and deformable, i.e. *plastic*, before they change state into a hard rigid mass. The change of state is usually as a result of a setting reaction. The resultant rigid restoration is often brittle and non-adhesive. Most restorations are made with this group of materials because the materials can be easily managed in the dental surgery, do not require extra stages and laboratory facilities, and are less expensive than those materials which are rigid on insertion.

The plastic materials may be considered in three groups: amalgam, resins and cements. A brief description is given but reference should be made to a textbook on dental materials for further information.

7.2 Amalgam

This is the most widely used restorative material, particularly in posterior teeth. Its formulation has not changed markedly since the turn of the century, which is more a reflection that no other material has better properties than that amalgam is ideal. Its major failings are a colour dissimilar to enamel and a lack of adhesion. Amalgam has a good shelf-life, is comparatively inexpensive and it can be mishandled to some extent without the end result being unacceptable. Amalgam restorations performed by a good operator in the right environment are long-lasting, but the average life in clinical practice is only 5 years.

Dental amalgam is made by mixing a silver–tin alloy with mercury; the resultant new alloy forms a very stiff paste which can be inserted into the cavity before it hardens.

The silver–tin alloy usually contains these metals in an approximate ratio of $3:1$ and is presented as a fine powder, which is mixed with a similar weight of liquid mercury to form two reaction products. The process may be represented as:

$$Ag_3Sn + Hg \rightarrow Ag_2Hg_3 + Sn_7Hg$$
$$\quad\; \gamma \qquad\qquad\quad \gamma_1 \qquad\; \gamma_2$$

The mercury only reacts with the atoms on the surface of the alloy particles to produce a thin coating of reaction products which bind together the cores of the original particles in the set amalgam. No free mercury remains. The set amalgam thus consists of particles of unreacted silver–tin alloy (γ) held in a matrix of the new γ_1 and γ_2 phases.

The tin phase (γ_2) is regarded as the less desirable of the reaction products because it is considered to increase corrosion and reduce the strength of the set amalgam. As the γ_2 and γ_1 contents of amalgam are directly related, the only practical way of reducing the amount of γ_2 is to produce an amalgam with as little matrix as possible and this is achieved by mixing a minimal amount of mercury with the original alloy; and the mixed amalgam should be compressed into the cavity so that the unreacted cores of the γ particles are packed closely together, with the surplus mercury-rich material being brought to the surface as a layer of excess material, which is then removed.

The search for a better amalgam has led the manufacturers in recent years to develop alloys which, when mixed with mercury, have little or no γ_2 content. These alloys contain a significant amount of copper (often 12% or more); this has been achieved by a reduction in the amount of silver. The copper is present either as part of the silver–tin alloy, making a single silver–tin–copper alloy, or is introduced (admixed) as separate particles of silver–copper alloy. In either case when the alloy reacts with mercury a copper–tin reaction product (η phase) is formed in preference to γ_2:

$$Ag\text{–}Sn\text{–}Cu + Hg \rightarrow \underset{\gamma_1}{Ag_2Hg_3} + \underset{\eta}{Cu_6Sn_5}$$

These newer amalgams corrode less and have greater marginal integrity than amalgams from conventional alloys. The physical form of the high copper alloy which is mixed with mercury appears to have little effect on the properties of the resultant amalgam.

For many years amalgam alloys have been produced by forming a molten alloy of the desired constituents, allowing it to soldify into a bar, then turning it on a lathe to produce small particles which are collected, ground and heat-treated. By adding a trace (1%) of zinc to the molten alloy, the other metals do not become oxidized during the manufacturing process. The particles are rough and of variable size which is controlled by the manufacturer (Fig. 7.1, *left*).

More recently, spherical alloys have been produced by atomizing the molten metal into an inert gas. With the possibility of oxidation eliminated, these alloys do not contain zinc. Spherical particles have the smallest surface area and so spherical alloys react with the least amount of mercury; they are also considerably easier to pack into a cavity as the spheres readily slide over each other. An alloy composed entirely of spherical particles is shown in Fig. 7.1 (*middle*), while a mixed alloy is shown in Fig. 7.1 (*right*).

PRESENTATION OF AMALGAM

The powdered alloy is supplied in a variety of forms: as loose powder sold by weight in glass bottles, as pellets of compressed powder or in disposable capsules ready for mixing. Mercury is supplied either in unbreakable bottles or in disposable capsules with the alloy. Mercury may present a hazard in the dental surgery, particularly when being dispensed or transferred from one container to another.

100 μm

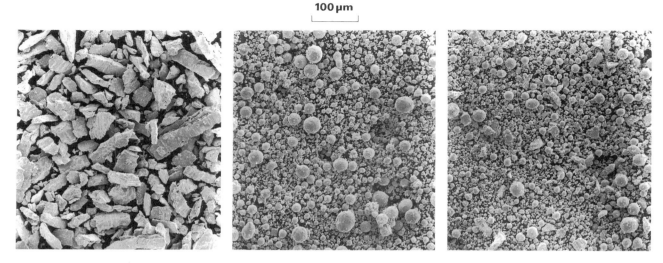

Fig. 7.1 *Left*: Scanning electron micrograph of lathecut particles of amalgam alloy. *Middle*: Scanning electron micrograph of spherical particles of amalgam alloy. *Right*: Scanning electron micrograph of mixed spherical and lathecut particles of amalgam alloy. Magnification of all parts × 130.

MERCURY HAZARDS

The vapour from uncombined mercury can present a toxic hazard to the dentist and DSA, but when it is combined, as in amalgam restorations, it is non-toxic. To reduce this hazard, mercury should always be stored in sealed containers away from heat. When it is dispensed into the reservoir of a mixing machine, the procedure should always be done over a tray to collect any mercury that might be spilled. Spilled mercury must always be cleaned up immediately and stored under water in a sealed container along with waste amalgam. If the spilled mercury is visible and accessible it should be collected together using a piece of card and then drawn into a one-piece disposable plastic pipette for transfer to the waste amalgam container. This method is preferable to using lead foil from X-ray film packets, for although the mercury combines with the lead, the contaminated lead foil must then be disposed of safely. Large spillages for which all the mercury cannot be accounted should be brought to the attention of the dentist responsible for the surgery and the local office of the Health and Safety Executive. The use of a mixture of sulphur and lime is of no value. Mercury is a highly reactive metal so it should not be allowed to contact gold and silver jewellery or metal waste pipes from sinks.

The use of disposable capsules which contain precise amounts of alloy and mercury fixed by the manufacturer eliminates the need to handle mercury in the dental surgery; once used the capsule should be reassembled and disposed; it should not be reused. Whenever amalgam is used, a small amount of vapour will be emitted and this should be removed by efficient ventilation of the surgery.

Recommendations on the handling of mercury have been produced by the American Dental Association (1976).

In recent years, there has been concern about the toxicity of amalgam restorations, and as a result some patients have requested replacement of all their amalgam fillings by tooth-coloured materials. The subject was reviewed by Eley and Cox (1987) who found a lack of evidence to condemn such a widely used dental material.

PROPORTIONING

The exact proportion of alloy to mercury will depend on both the alloy and the mixing technique being used; in the case of disposable capsules this has been determined by the manufacturer. In general, if too little mercury were used there would be insufficient to coat the surface of all the particles, and this would result in a 'dry' mix. This dry paste would be difficult to manipulate and inevitably result in a porous restoration of low strength. If too much mercury was mixed with the alloy, a 'wet' mix would result; it would be difficult to compress the wet paste into the cavity in the tooth because of the presence of a mercury-rich layer at the surface. The amalgam would also take longer to set and in the case of amalgam using conventional alloy it is likely that the restoration would have a high γ_2 content, causing decreased strength and increased corrosion.

Disposable capsules are accurate and quick, but inevitably expensive. They provide convenience, and waste is kept to a minimum.

Bulk dispenser/mixers are widely used, and are normally accurate and quick. They require periodic maintenance and work best with lathe-cut alloys. Care must be taken to avoid spillage when filling the reservoir with mercury. The unit cost of amalgam is lower than using disposable capsules.

MIXING

Thorough mixing is necessary to produce an amalgam which can be manipulated easily. It is now universally achieved with a mixing machine which oscillates a small capsule. Some machines accept a disposable capsule into spring-loaded arms (Fig. 7.2) and can produce

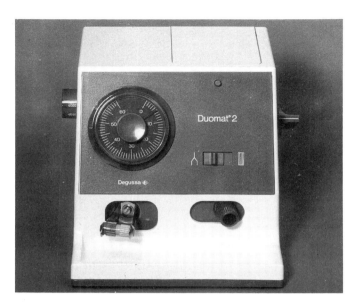

Fig. 7.2 A machine for mixing amalgam, either by oscillating a disposable capsule (*left*), or by oscillating amalgam alloy and mercury dispensed into the reusable capsule (*right*) from the reservoirs inside. The length of mixing is varied by the timer.

an amalgam within 5 seconds. Others which also dispense the alloy and mercury have a reusable capsule (Fig. 7.2) and take a little longer (20 seconds). The amalgam should be mixed for the time recommended by the manufacturer of the alloy for the machine in use. After it has been mixed, the amalgam paste should have a smooth, very stiff consistency.

The amalgam should be inserted into the tooth before it sets, as once crystallization has begun, manipulation becomes difficult and, if continued, would cause a reduction in the strength of the amalgam. The working time depends on the type of alloy and method of mixing, and can range from 3 to 10 minutes. The shorter working time suits the busy practitioner because time is not wasted waiting for crystallization to occur; in addition, matrix bands may be removed sooner with less chance of damage to the restoration, and checking of occlusal contacts is unlikely to be accompanied by fracture of the amalgam. The longer working time suits the inexperienced operator, particularly with large restorations, because he has time to pack the amalgam, carve away any gingival overhangs of amalgam and check occlusal contacts before the amalgam becomes too hard to carve. On setting, amalgam contracts by about 0.05%; the exact dimensional change is dependent on the alloy and type and length of mixing. When mixing was formerly done by hand, there was often a small expansion.

STRENGTH

For restorations in amalgam to be successful, they must be strong enough to resist masticatory forces. Additional strength is of little clinical value, so the absolute strength is unimportant as long as it meets or exceeds national or international standards. The way that the amalgam is handled is likely to be far more significant, since a porous amalgam is weak and liable to fracture.

Amalgam takes some hours to reach full hardness and when fully set its compressive strength is similar to dentine. Amalgam is weak in thin section and fractures in a brittle manner. Its strengths after 24 hours are given in Table 7.1. Manufacturers often quote the 1-hour strength, which gives an indication of the rate of hardening of the amalgam. High early strength implies a fast setting amalgam which means that there is a short working time for the operator.

Table 7.1 24-hour strength of a typical amalgam.

Strength	MN/m^2
Compressive	320
Tensile	55

MOISTURE CONTAMINATION

Contamination of the amalgam with water or blood during insertion of the restoration is detrimental and accelerates corrosion, particularly if the alloy contains zinc because hydrogen gas is formed, producing a porous restoration and excessive expansion which could cause pain. It is therefore very important to keep the cavity dry during insertion of amalgam.

CORROSION

Amalgam is liable to corrode, particularly in the environmental conditions of the mouth because of its heterogeneous structure, rough surface and incomplete oxide film. Tin from the γ_2 phase is the element that most readily passes into solution to form an unstable oxide film on the surface. In common with rusting of ferrous materials there is

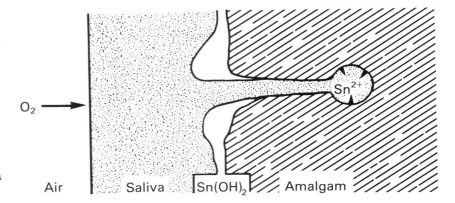

Fig. 7.3 Diagram of pitting corrosion of amalgam. Tin passes into solution and forms an unstable oxide on the surface where it combines with oxygen.

deep pitting corrosion, which if allowed to continue cannot be eliminated by polishing. Pitting corrosion is shown diagrammatically in Fig. 7.3.

A poorly compressed amalgam restoration which is porous is very susceptible to corrosion. The accessible surfaces of the restoration should be polished a few days after insertion to make them smooth with a passive oxide layer that resists corrosion. The surfaces in contact with the cavity walls are also susceptible to corrosion; but the process may be partly self-limiting on the deeper surfaces because of the accumulation of mineral deposits from saliva or corrosion products. Corrosion on these surfaces may be reduced to some extent by coating the walls of the cavity with varnish prior to insertion of the amalgam. In the long term this corrosion results in the migration of tin ions into the enamel and dentine, which then appear more blue than normal. Mechanical stress is known to accelerate corrosion; and marginal breakdown, usually known as ditching, is considered to be caused by corrosion. The more recently introduced high-copper amalgams corrode noticeably less because of the virtual absence of γ_2 and they demonstrate substantially reduced marginal breakdown.

ADHESION AND BIOCOMPATIBILITY

Amalgam has no adhesion to enamel or dentine. There is therefore a potential microspace between any restoration and tooth. Microleakage may be reduced in the early life of the restoration by coating the cavity walls with varnish. After a few months, microleakage of a restoration in an unvarnished cavity is reduced by mineral deposits from saliva or corrosion products at the interface.

Amalgam is regarded as being non-irritant but the failure of the material to bond to the tooth allows oral bacteria to pass round the restoration and irritate the pulp through the dentinal tubules. For this reason the walls of the cavity against the pulp should be covered with a lining material, and the remaining walls coated with varnish.

7.3   Composite resins

Restorative materials based on the polymerization of organic resins have been used in anterior teeth since the late 1940s, but substantial modifications have occurred during the intervening period. When resins were first introduced as restorative materials, methyl methacrylate resin was used on its own; subsequently the resin was filled with an inorganic filler. The most significant change came with the switch from an aliphatic to an aromatic dimethacrylate resin and coating of the filler particles with a silane coupling agent which binds the filler to the resin. Every development has been heralded as a major breakthrough but even now the ultimate material has not arrived.

The present generation of composite resins was introduced in the late 1960s, and has become the most widely used restorative material for anterior teeth, because it is easy to use, has a good colour match and its mechanical properties are better than those of any alternative. Since the late 1960s changes in composition and developments in chemical formulation have been relatively small. The earlier materials were autopolymerizing; however, current materials are now polymerized by intense white light. The resin is based on BIS-GMA, the reaction product of bisphenol A and glycidyl methacrylate, to which are added more volatile monomers such as triethylene glycol dimethacrylate (TEDMA) or, less commonly, methyl methacrylate to act as diluents. The composite resin contains inorganic fillers, such as quartz on silicate glass, which are organosilane-coated to allow bonding between the resin and filler.

TYPES OF COMPOSITE RESIN

Composite resins now available may be divided into different types according to their filler loading (Table 7.2).

The search for more durable composite resins than the original conventional ones has resulted in development in two different directions. One avenue has been to reduce the size of the filler particles to an average size of 0.04 μm. However, the percentage of filler is much lower by weight (52%). This has produced a material which can be polished but is more prone to wear; two examples are Helio Progress (Vivadent, Liechtenstein) and Silux (3M Health Care, Loughborough,

Table 7.2 Classification of composite resins.

	Average particle size (μm)	Filter	
		Weight	Volume
Conventional	11	78	64
Microfilled	0.04	52	27
Hybrid	8	77	63
Posterior	3	85	74

Leicestershire). In order to overcome the low abrasion resistance, manufacturers have produced 'hybrid' materials which contain both conventional filler particles and the submicron particles; an example is Prismafil (Dentsply, Weybridge, Surrey).

The other avenue has been to increase the total filler content with particles of various sizes so that the amount of resin is very low; an example is P-50 (3M Health Care, Loughborough, Leicestershire). With far less resin to wear preferentially, abrasion is resisted; this type of material is intended for posterior teeth and is still being developed, although a recent 5-year clinical trial of a comparable material has reported little deterioration in the restorations over the period. Composite resins for posterior teeth are normally radiopaque so that the restorations may be distinguished from dental caries.

PRESENTATION

Composite resin filling material is usually presented as a paste in a light-proof syringe (Fig. 7.4). The material is polymerized by intense visible light (wavelength approximately 470 nm). The operator has time to dispense the material, place it in the cavity and adapt any matrix strip before curing the composite resin for 20–60 seconds. The longer time is required for thick layers, dark shades and highly filled

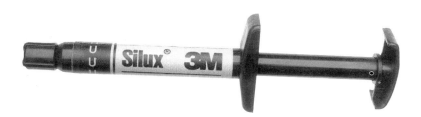

Fig. 7.4 An example of a syringe of a light-cured composite resin, which is kept in a light-proof container.

resins (e.g. posterior composite resin). If the curing time is too short, the surface of the restoration may be hard but the bottom will be 'soggy', causing premature failure. Where the restoration is large (>4 mm thick) it is better to insert and cure the material in increments, and to apply the light in different places. The light must be placed as close as possible to the composite resin. Curing in increments also helps to reduce setting contraction.

Previously, composite resin was supplied as two pastes which were identical except that one contained an accelerator while the other contained the initiator together with an inhibitor to prevent premature setting. When similar amounts of each paste were thoroughly mixed, polymerization was initiated. The operator had several minutes to manipulate the material before it rapidly set hard, although further polymerization continued for some hours. The mixing of two pastes caused air entrapment, and this porosity contributed to discoloration of the material after a period in the mouth.

Another defunct method of polymerizing composite resin was by ultraviolet light, but this method was discontinued because of the possible harm to patient, dentist and his DSA.

COLOUR

The composite resins have a high degree of translucency, and their colour is dependent on the type and particle size of the filler chosen by the manufacturer and added colouring, since the resin is virtually transparent. The filler contributes colour by light reflection and dispersion, which usually allows the restoration to assume the colour of the tooth and appear imperceptible to the casual eye. Since BIS-GMA composite resins were introduced, the average size of filler particles has been lowered to reduce roughness on the surface of restorations. For the majority of patients a universal-shade paste is suitable, but to match teeth whose colour is outside the normal range, specially pigmented pastes may be used.

In the long term, restorations made from light-cured composite resin maintain colour well; however, those from a two-paste composite resin may discolour because of the effect of the chemical initiator, usually benzoyl peroxide.

STRENGTH AND WEAR

The tensile and compressive strengths are not as high as amalgam and are given in Table 7.3. The tensile strength and fracture toughness are sufficiently high to allow composite resins to be used for the restora-

Table 7.3 Strength of composite resin.

Strength	Hybrid (MN/m^2)	Posterior (MN/m^2)
Compressive	240	300
Tensile	40	54

tion of incisal angles; this extends their clinical application compared with glass ionomer cement. When composite resin materials were first introduced, it was considered that they would have adequate strength to be used on the occlusal surfaces of posterior teeth. What had not been predicted was the unacceptably high wear that occurred, because the resin was preferentially worn away around the filler particles which then became undermined and dislodged. Therefore, conventional composite resin materials have not been endorsed for restoring occlusal surfaces of posterior teeth; however, specific posterior materials have been developed and these show a much more acceptable rate of wear, similar to amalgam.

Wear of conventional composite resin by the trimming process caused a rough surface which readily stained, particularly in patients who smoked. The surface was not amenable to polishing. The surface of posterior composite resin is less rough, but the smoothest surface which can be polished after trimming is found with the microfilled composite resins.

SETTING

From the clinical aspect, setting of light-cured material occurs within a few seconds of applying the light and setting of a two-paste composite resin occurs within a few minutes of mixing. Once set, the composite resin cannot be carved with sharp hand instruments as can amalgam or some glass ionomer cements; instead the use of rotary abrasives is required. Compared with the unfilled methyl methacrylate resins, which were at one time used as restorative materials, the composite resins have an appreciably lower exotherm, smaller setting contraction and lower coefficient of thermal expansion.

ADHESION

Composite resins themselves do not bond chemically to enamel, but two clinical methods of bonding are used. First, there is physical bonding, which is now widely used. It is possible to etch enamel to create selective pores into which the unset resin can flow and polymerize; this mechanical locking gives very good retention. The use of etched enamel for retention is unique to resin-based restorative materials and has enabled these materials to be used in situations where conventional forms of retention would be unavailable or unsuitable. It has also been employed to eliminate marginal staining around composite resin restorations and to provide a seal. To ensure good contact between the etched enamel and composite resin, a number of manufacturers recommend that a low viscosity resin (the composite resin without filler) should be applied to the etched enamel before the composite resin. Research has shown that this is not absolutely necessary, but clinically the operator is more sure of achieving an effective bond by its use.

Second, the use of an intermediate layer of a dentine bonding agent to bond a resin-based restorative material to dentine has been investigated by a number of workers over many years. However, because a lining is placed over the pulpal wall of the cavity, the available area of dentine for bonding is small. Several manufacturers have produced dentine bonding agents based on phosphorus esters of BIS-GMA and more recently have used hydrophylic coupling resins (hydroxyethyl methylmethacrylate), which appear to be the most favourable yet investigated as regards both bonding and biocompatibility; the bonding to dentine *in vitro* is better than that of glass ionomer cement; however, it may decrease with time *in vivo* as hydrolysis of the bonding agent occurs. An example of the most recent type of dentine bonding agent is Scotchbond 2 (3M Health Care, Loughborough, Leicestershire).

STORAGE

Composite resin restorative materials have a limited shelf-life (approximately 1–2 years) which may be prolonged by refrigeration. The material should be stored in a cool dark place, and it is essential that the cap is replaced on the syringe, or lid on the container.

BIOCOMPATIBILITY

Composite resin restorative materials have been regarded as being irritant to the pulp when placed in unlined cavities. However, it has been shown by a number of workers, in particular Brännström, that the pulpal irritation is caused by the bacteria and their toxins which colonize the microspace between the restoration and the cavity wall. To prevent pulpal damage, the dentine walls of the cavity should be lined with a suitable lining cement and the acid-etch technique should be used on the peripheral enamel to obtain mechanical bonding of the restoration.

7.4 Cements

Cements based on the reaction between a silicate glass and an acid have been used in dentistry for 100 years. They are of a similar colour to tooth and are suitable for some restorations in anterior teeth. Their low tensile strength and brittleness have prevented their use for restoring incisal angles of anterior teeth and the occlusal surfaces of posterior teeth. The cements are prone to dissolution by acids from overlying plaque. Until the development of glass ionomer cement by Wilson & Kent (1972), silicate cement was widely used almost as the sole plastic anterior filling material. Shortly before glass ionomer cement was introduced, composite resins were developed such that they became the most widely used anterior filling materials. Nevertheless, the use of glass ionomer cement has increased particularly because it adheres to dentine and to enamel; since the cement's initial introduction it has become available in types which are quicker setting, less soluble, more translucent and aesthetically acceptable.

SILICATE CEMENT

Silicate cement is so little used that its properties and handling will not be considered further; the interested reader should refer to the review by Wilson (1975).

GLASS IONOMER CEMENT

Essentially, glass ionomer cement is formed by reacting a specially prepared alumino-silicate glass with polyacrylic acid. After being mixed, the cement paste is inserted into the cavity before it hardens.

The setting reaction has similarities with that of amalgam, in that the acid only reacts with the surface of the glass particles to form a thin coating of cement which binds together the cores of unreacted glass (Fig. 7.5). Initially a calcium salt is formed, but the calcium ions are subsequently replaced by aluminium ions to form a hard cement. Fluoride salts are released from the glass and these are considered to help prevent recurrent caries. The cement exhibits extensive cross-linking between chains because of the large molecular weight polyanion; this contributes to the cement's ability to resist dissolution under acidic conditions.

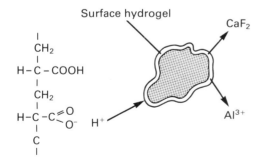

Fig. 7.5 The setting reaction of glass ionomer cement; the acid attacks the glass particles to form a surface hydrogel with release of calcium and aluminium ions. The aluminium ions form a cross-linked structure with the acid polyanion.

The original cements were slow to set, prone to moisture contamination immediately after setting and had a poor appearance because of poor translucency. The manufacturers have now developed the cements so that they are easier to mix, set more quickly, are therefore less prone to moisture contamination and have improved appearance. Some are now radiopaque.

The glass : acid ratio is important for development of a cement with desirable physical properties. To overcome the variability of mixing the cement on a glass slab, some manufacturers have produced a powder containing the glass and dried polyacrylic acid in optimal proportions; the operator just adds water to initiate the setting reaction. Manufacturers have also produced the cement in capsule form to overcome the errors of hand dispensing and mixing.

Glass ionomer cement containing silver fused in the glass has been developed, and is known by the generic name of cermet. It has improved abrasion resistance and is radiopaque; it has therefore been used in posterior teeth but in relatively protected cavities since it is not as strong as amalgam.

Specially formulated versions of the cement have been produced as lining cements and luting cements (page 144). Most recently a lining cement has been produced, the setting reaction of which is accelerated by the application of intense white light. Glass ionomer cements have been reviewed by McLean (1988).

ADHESION

A property unique to glass ionomer cements is the ability to bond chemically with both dentine and enamel. Extensive use of this has been made in the restoration of cervical abrasions without the need for any cavity preparation; these are situations where there is very little, if any, enamel for retention of composite resin. The cement may be used as the sole restorative material or it may be used as a base and veneered with composite resin.

BIOCOMPATIBILITY

Although glass ionomer cement can be placed in deep cavities without causing pulpal irritation even when no cavity lining is used, it is advisable to place a lining in cavities with a large number of freshly cut dentinal tubules to prevent any reaction. The generally minimal reaction of the pulp would appear to result from the cement's adhesion to enamel and dentine preventing bacterial leakage. The high biocompatibility occurs despite the freshly mixed cement being very acidic; however, severe inflammation can occur if the cement is applied directly to a pulpal exposure.

MOISTURE CONTAMINATION

Contamination of the cement with saliva during insertion into the cavity and before it has completely set is very detrimental: the restoration is likely to dissolve and adhesion is reduced. It is most important that the cavity is kept dry by effective isolation during insertion of the material and also that the restoration is covered by an impervious layer of polymerized resin or varnish during the subsequent few hours to prevent desiccation by water loss or dissolution by water gain.

Bibliography

American Dental Association (1976) Recommendations in mercury hygiene. *Journal of the American Dental Association*, **92**, 1217.

Brännström M. (1984) Communication between the oral cavity and the dental pulp associated with restorative treatment. *Operative Dentistry*, **9**, 57–68.

Brännström M. & Nordenvall K. J. (1978) Bacterial penetration, pulpal reaction and the inner surface of Concise Enamel Bond. Composite fillings in etched and unetched cavities. *Journal of Dental Research*, **57**, 3–10.

Brown D. (1988) Dental amalgam. *British Dental Journal*, **164**, 253–256.

Combe E. C. (1986) *Notes on Dental Materials*, 5th edn. Churchill Livingstone, Edinburgh.

Craig R. G. (1981) Chemistry, composition and properties of composite resins. *Dental Clinics of North America*, **25**, 219–239.

Craig R. G. (1989) *Restorative Dental Materials*, 8th edn. Mosby, St. Louis.

Eley B. M. & Cox S. W. (1987) Mercury from dental amalgam fillings in patients. *British Dental Journal*, **163**, 221–226.

McCabe J. F. (1985) *Anderson's Applied Dental Materials*, 6th edn. Blackwell Scientific Publications, Oxford.

McLean J. W. (1988) Glass-ionomer cements. *British Dental Journal*, **164**, 293–300.

Robinson A. A., Rowe A. H. R. & Maberley M. L. (1988) A three-year study of the clinical performance of a posterior composite and a lathe cut amalgam alloy. *British Dental Journal*, **164**, 248–252.

Wilson A. D. (1975) Dental cements based on ion-leachable glasses. In von Fraunhofer J. A. (ed.) *Scientific Aspects of Dental Materials*, pp. 191–221. Butterworth, London.

Wilson A. D. & Kent B. E. (1972) A new translucent cement for dentistry. The glass ionomer cement. *British Dental Journal*, **132**, 133–135.

Wilson A. D. & McLean J. W. (1988) *Glass-ionomer Cement*. Quintessence, Chicago.

Wilson N. H. F., Wilson M. A., Wastell D. G. & Smith G. A. (1988) A clinical trial of a visible light cured posterior composite resin restorative material: five-year results. *Quintessence International*, **19**, 675–681.

8 Preparations for plastic restorative materials

8.1 Introduction

The principles of cavity preparation for all the plastic restorative materials are generally similar because cavity form is largely determined by removal of carious enamel and dentine, and therefore cavities for these materials are considered in one section. Cavities in posterior teeth, being more common, will be covered first, and simpler cavities will be discussed before the more complex. The description of cavities will usually be related to specific examples with emphasis on principles for individual application.

8.2 Occlusal cavity

SMALL OCCLUSAL CAVITY

A small carious lesion in the fissure system of an upper premolar will be considered first. In the mesial pit there is staining of the enamel but there is neither visible cavitation nor discoloration of the dentine visible through the enamel surrounding the pit. There is also no evidence on a bitewing radiograph of occlusal caries. The patient has also had a higher than average prevalence of caries for children of his age, and the tooth has only been erupted for 1–2 years.

Management should consist of:

1 dietary advice,
2 investigation of the carious lesion,
3 fissure sealing.

When a small restoration is combined with fissure sealing, the procedure is referred to as a *preventive resin restoration* (Simonsen 1980) or a *sealant restoration*, and this procedure has now gained clinical acceptance.

It is essential that the preventive resin restoration is placed under effective isolation from salivary contamination, and it is therefore most convenient to perform the whole procedure under rubber dam isolation (page 253).

The first stage of cavity preparation is access to the carious enamel and dentine; this is achieved with a small round bur (ISO size 008 or 010) in the turbine handpiece. The fast running bur is slowly inserted to the depth of its cutting head or slightly more (up to 1.5 mm), with the operator ensuring that there is adequate water cooling. The bur is then withdrawn from the tooth, which is dried for visual examination of the presence of carious enamel on each wall and carious dentine on the floor. The sites where further removal of carious tooth structure is required should be noted. The bur is then reinserted into the cavity to remove the carious tissue. The cavity is redried to see if all the carious enamel and dentine has been removed; should any remain, it is removed. No attempt is made to cut a cavity with a preconceived outline or cross-section. Only carious tooth structure and the smallest amount of enamel to achieve access should have been drilled away. The enamel margins should be planed with a sharp chisel to remove any unsupported prisms. Cavity preparation for the preventive resin restoration is now complete and insertion of the restoration is covered on page 130.

LARGE OCCLUSAL CAVITY

In the centre of the occlusal surface of a lower second molar, a carious lesion that has advanced to the stage where the enamel walls of the central fossa appear demineralized clinically and where discoloration of the dentine may be seen through the surrounding enamel will be considered. A radiolucency is visible in the dentine beneath the occlusal enamel on a bitewing radiograph. There will be bacterial penetration of the underlying dentine and the lesion is in need of treatment; in this example, caries involving dentine is not considered to be present in the four extensions of the fissure (Fig. 8.1). The most efficient method of working is to use rubber dam isolation for preparation and restoration (page 253). Since the restoration is in a molar and will be exposed to occlusal wear, it is planned to use amalgam.

The first stage of cavity preparation is access to the carious dentine; this is achieved by use of a small round or pear-shaped bur (ISO size 008 or 010) in the turbine handpiece.

It has been usual practice to include all the fissures on the occlusal surface within the outline of the cavity unless there is a specific reason to the contrary, such as a low rate of caries and no evidence of caries extending in the fissures; this aspect has been considered on page 69. The cavity should be kept as small as possible, commensurate with removing carious dentine. Where doubt exists about the extent of caries at this stage, it is better to create a small cavity, for it can always be enlarged after reaching dentine but not vice versa.

Having decided the extent of the cavity along the fissures, the operator should place a thin bur (ISO size 008) in the turbine handpiece, because a thin bur allows the width of the cavity extensions along the fissures to be kept narrow. The shape of bur used to prepare

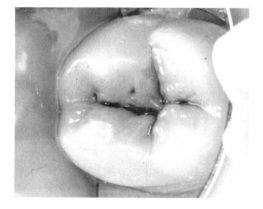

Fig. 8.1 Occlusal caries in a lower left second molar.

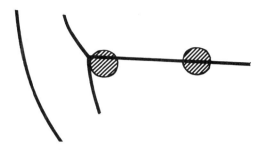

Fig. 8.2 During preparation of the main fissure the bur is centred on the fissure, but close to the marginal ridge it is kept towards the bulk of the tooth.

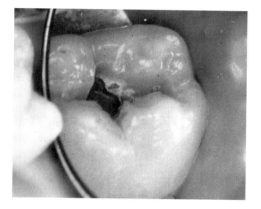

Fig. 8.3 Carious enamel (white) is present on one wall. Carious dentine is present on the floor (dark).

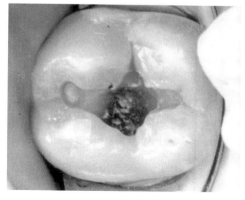

Fig. 8.4 Caries only now remains in dentine in the centre of the cavity floor.

the cavity is important: the preferred bur is pear-shaped because it cuts well both on its side and on its end, but does not overenlarge the cavity. The alternative use of a round bur is mainly suited to small cavities; the use of a small round bur to extend fissures in a large cavity is unduly tedious and the desired shape may also be more difficult to create. Plain fissure burs which were once favoured are now considered to give too much geometrical shape to the cavity. Inverted cone burs are unsuitable because they readily create unsupported enamel and undermine the marginal ridges. With any type of bur the surface outline of the cavity has rounded angles which facilitate subsequent insertion of amalgam. The bur is then moved across the entire extent of the fissure that is to be treated, removing a thin layer of enamel. By making a shallow cut over a large area, the waterspray is unlikely to be obstructed in contrast to deep penetration of the bur, and this should avoid any overheating of the tooth. With the main fissures the bur is centred on the fissure, but at the mesial and distal ends where the fissure may fork, the bur is kept towards the bulk of the tooth to avoid weakening the marginal ridges of enamel (Fig. 8.2). The handpiece is lowered a little more and the entire cavity deepened. Gradually, cavity depth is increased until the amelo-dentinal junction is just penetrated. At this stage the width of the fissure extensions is very slightly greater than the diameter of the thin bur used. The long axis of the bur throughout preparation should be held approximately perpendicular to the occlusal surface.

Drilling should stop on reaching the amelo-dentinal junction to allow the cavity to be dried and examined for caries both at the amelo-dentinal junction and on the pulpal floor. In this example, carious enamel is present on one wall, and carious dentine is found in the central fossa area both at the amelo-dentinal junction and on the cavity floor (Fig 8.3) but none is found in the fissure extensions. The carious dentine feels softer to the point of a probe than sound dentine and is usually a darker colour.

The cavity should only be widened more where there is enamel caries and dentinal caries at the amelo-dentinal junction, using the turbine bur inserted to the full depth of the cavity. No more widening should be done than is necessary to remove carious dentine at the amelo-dentinal junction; overhanging enamel must be taken away as it is brittle and if allowed to remain would fracture subsequently. The carious dentine in the centre of the cavity floor will still remain and is *not* removed at this stage. The cavity prepared so far is shown in Fig. 8.4.

Resistance to dislodgement of the restoration is provided by the cavity shape which has already been prepared, i.e. a cavity floor in the

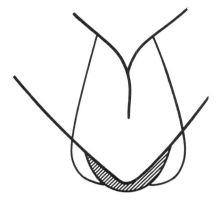

Fig. 8.5 Outline of cavity superimposed on cross-section of a fissure. The cavity floor is in approximately the same plane as the occlusal surface for resistance to displacement of the restoration. The walls converge occlusally for retention. The hatched area indicates carious dentine.

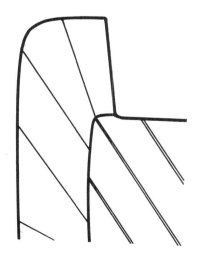

Fig. 8.6 The marginal ridge must not be undermined.

same plane as the occlusal surface and cavity walls which are approximately perpendicular to the floor (Fig. 8.5).

Retention is gained by minimal convergence of the cavity walls (Fig. 8.5); this is achieved by a pear-shaped bur or by slight angulation of a fissure bur. Most operators create retentive form while cavity extension is being carried out rather than at a separate stage. The cavity should be examined after the amelo-dentinal junction is caries-free to assess retention. The mesial and distal walls of the cavity are not angled to provide retention because in doing so the marginal ridges would be undesirably weakened (Fig. 8.6). As the cavity has been prepared only just into dentine, the cavity is widest at the amelo-dentinal junction.

The enamel margins should now be smoothed to remove unsupported prisms which exist after the use of burs. This is best achieved using binangled and hatchet chisels, the choice of which depends on site and access. The cavo-surface angle will vary depending on its position, but should never be less than a right angle, otherwise there would be unsupported enamel prisms. On a steep cusp it may be as high as 120°, and some operators prefer to reduce this nearer to 90° to increase the margin angle of amalgam; this may be achieved by altering the angle of the bur and drilling only the superficial part of the enamel (Fig. 8.7). Unsupported enamel will not occur provided that the cavo-surface angle remains greater than 90°. There is no need to extend the widening of the cavity to its floor; indeed, such tooth removal is unnecessary and undesirable.

By this stage, carious dentine will remain only in the central part of the pulpal floor and, being much softer than sound dentine, can be readily detected with the tip of an excavator. To make it visible to the operator, a small pledget of cotton wool soaked in 1% Acid Red dye in propanol should be placed on the cavity floor to stain the carious dentine bright red. The operator aims to remove solely carious dentine using a medium-sized round bur (ISO size 012) in the low-speed handpiece, which gives the operator much greater feel in the removal of carious dentine than does a turbine handpiece. The use of waterspray is very valuable because it washes away the chips of carious dentine and enables the operator to see the surface being cut; the speed of the bur is not critical but is often in the range 1000–8000 r.p.m. With the extent of lesion present in this example, it should be possible to remove the softened dentine completely without exposing the pulp by a gentle painting action with the bur; pressure should not be applied to the bur. The translucent hypermineralized zone, by virtue of its hardness, should make a very convenient limit to cavity depth. If the deepest part of the cavity floor appears dark but feels hard, this may

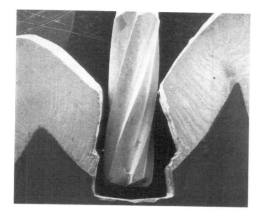

Fig. 8.7 Scanning electron micrograph of a bur placed in a cavity (longitudinal section, magnification × 11). The cavo-surface angles have been altered on the steep cusp slopes to increase the margin angles of the restoration.

not be carious dentine but could be hypermineralized dentine or even reactionary dentine which has formed in response to caries. The hard stained dentine should not be removed because pulpal damage or exposure could easily occur. If any red-stained dentine remains, it should be removed with the bur.

Had the lesion been more extensive, then it is possible that removal of all the softened dentine on the cavity floor would result in pulpal exposure which is undesirable. Therefore, in a symptomless tooth without signs of irreversible pulpitis a trace of softened non-stained dentine would be left; this remaining demineralized dentine caries rarely continues to spread provided that a satisfactory restoration is placed. Some operators prefer to remove carious dentine with excavators, but inexperienced operators will find them less easy to control and more time-consuming to use than burs.

After the removal of carious dentine in the central part of the cavity, the cavity floor will be at two levels, and it should be left like this (Fig. 8.8). There is no value in deepening the shallow part of the floor; in fact a great deal of pulpal damage would result by the removal of more sound dentine and the tooth would be significantly weakened.

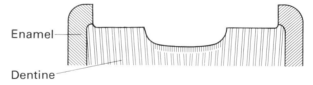

Enamel

Dentine

Fig. 8.8 Diagram of the cavity floor after caries removal in the central region of a lower molar (longitudinal mesio-distal section).

The cavity is washed with the waterspray from the 3-in-1 syringe and then dried gently with compressed air. The cavity should be examined from various aspects to ensure that carious dentine has been completely removed from the entire amelo-dentinal junction and that the cavity will be retentive, i.e. undercut (Fig. 8.9). It is then ready for inserting the restoration (page 118).

Some authorities in the past have suggested that the cavity width, bucco-lingually, should be one-third the intercuspal distance. There is no justification for such overenlargement routinely. The width of the cavity is governed by the size of the smallest bur available; it is only widened further to remove caries from the amelo-dentinal junction.

In the case of an upper molar where caries has affected both the central fossa and the distal fissure, the operator should treat the two lesions as separate entities, leaving the oblique ridge intact unless caries at the amelo-dentinal junction has undermined the ridge.

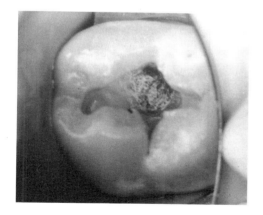

Fig. 8.9 The completed cavity in the lower second molar. No dye stained carious dentine remains on the cavity floor.

PIT CAVITY NOT ON THE OCCLUSAL SURFACE

Caries may occur in pits on the buccal surface of lower molars, the palatal surface of upper molars or the palatal surface of upper lateral incisors, and the disease can be well established before the teeth are fully erupted. In common with many carious pits, the extent of disease may be underestimated if the clinical examination is not thorough. The lesion should be treated in a similar way to a small carious pit on the occlusal surface of an upper premolar (page 91).

The cavity should be prepared with a small round bur in the turbine handpiece and the depth taken just into dentine. It is initially made about 1 mm in diameter and widened only by the presence of caries at the amelo-dentinal junction; caries governs the extent of the cavity. The small cavity may have slightly convergent enamel walls. In the larger cavity they may need to diverge to prevent leaving enamel prisms unsupported. A peripheral groove is created in dentine as a result of caries removal at the amelo-dentinal junction, and this provides retention.

Deep caries on the cavity floor is removed as the last stage of cavity preparation using a medium-sized round bur (ISO size 012) in the low-speed handpiece. In the past this type of cavity was usually restored with amalgam, but it is now more usual to use glass ionomer cement or composite resin.

CARIOUS FISSURE EXTENDING ONTO ANOTHER SURFACE

Some fissures extend onto a second surface of the tooth, the most frequent being the distal fissure of an upper molar extending onto the palatal surface and the occlusal fissure of a lower molar extending onto the buccal surface. The treatment of these fissures seems to confuse students and therefore needs some explanation.

If the distal fissure and palatal pit of an upper molar have each been affected by small carious lesions, then these should be treated as two separate single surface cavities with no intent of joining them. However, when the fissure between them is involved by caries, or both lesions are large, then a single cavity must be prepared. The width of the cavity in the fissure should be no wider than a thin fissure or pear-shaped bur (ISO size 008) unless the extent of caries at the amelo-dentinal junction causes it to be wider. The cavity depth should be just into dentine and only deepened further where carious dentine needs to be removed. The cavity depth should therefore be approximately constant from the tooth surface and about 2 mm deep (Fig. 8.10). Thus the operator needs to rotate the handpiece as the bur moves from the

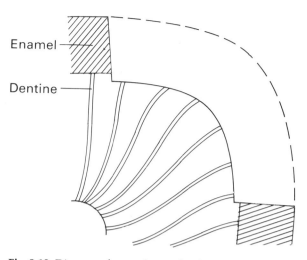

Enamel

Dentine

Fig. 8.10 Diagram of an occluso-palatal cavity showing how cavity depth is kept approximately constant by rotating the handpiece during preparation (longitudinal section).

occlusal to the palatal surface to ensure that the long axis of the bur stays perpendicular to the tooth surface. The enamel walls of a small cavity may converge slightly, providing retention, but should be stable because of prism angulation.

In the past, this type of cavity was restored with amalgam but it is now more usual to use glass ionomer cement or composite resin. In some instances a preventive resin restoration would be most appropriate.

8.3 Cervical cavity

In this example, caries has involved the enamel on the buccal surface of a lower molar in a band approximately 1 mm wide and cavitated in a limited area. Such a lesion develops because of poor plaque control and incorrect diet, and is really the only lesion that could have been prevented by adequate plaque control in the presence of incorrect diet. When cavitation of the enamel has occurred and bacteria have invaded the dentine, cavity preparation is almost always necessary. Very occasionally the lesion has become arrested; the affected tooth substance is darkly stained and it feels hard to a probe.

This type of cavity is best prepared with a small round bur because end-on access with fissure burs is often restricted by the head of the handpiece hitting the ascending ramus or cheek, or the coronoid process if an upper molar is being treated; in such circumstances a fissure

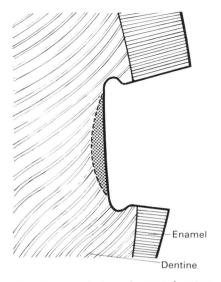

—Enamel

—Dentine

Fig. 8.11 Diagram of a buccal cavity showing retentive grooves occlusally and gingivally. The enamel walls should be flared to remove unsupported prisms. Carious dentine on the axial wall is indicated by stippling (longitudinal section).

bur might overcut the tooth. The initial cavity size is limited by the extent of carious enamel and the cavity depth should be taken just into dentine. This will reveal the extent of carious involvement of the amelo-dentinal junction. Further cavity preparation is done with the low-speed handpiece as the operator has more control and feel compared with the turbine handpiece. The cavity size should be enlarged until the amelo-dentinal junction is caries-free. Whilst the cavity depth occlusally should remain just into dentine, the depth gingivally should be not less than 1 mm from the tooth surface as the enamel, if present in this region, is invariably very thin. By this stage only carious dentine will remain on the wall of the cavity against the pulp (axial wall).

Retention should be provided by creating a small groove entirely in dentine along the occlusal and gingival walls using a small round bur (ISO size 008) in the low-speed handpiece (Fig. 8.11). In the process, unsupported enamel must not be created and it is for this reason that it is inappropriate to place retentive grooves on the mesial and distal walls of a wide cavity.

Next, the enamel walls should be smoothed with a binangled chisel to remove unsupported prisms; this will usually result in a flare to the occlusal and gingival walls (Fig. 8.11). The mesial and distal walls should be perpendicular to a tangent at the tooth surface.

The gingival wall should preferably be supragingival so that the plaque-accumulating margin of the restoration does not contribute to gingivitis. Its actual position will be dictated by the extent of caries at the amelo-dentinal junction.

The remaining stage is to remove caries from the affected part of the axial wall (Fig. 8.11) with a round bur (ISO size 012) in the low-speed handpiece. Removal of sound dentine from the axial wall is contra-indicated because the pulp is likely to be adversely affected since it is close.

The cavity should be washed and dried to check that the carious dentine has been removed and that sufficient retention has been provided for the restoration; the retentive grooves are of considerable importance for a restoration in amalgam, as the cavity is shallow. It is now usual for such a cavity to be restored with glass ionomer cement or composite resin; in the case of the latter material, a bevel is often placed on the occlusal margin with a fissure bur in the turbine handpiece to provide retention from etched enamel.

In older patients caries may occur at the neck of the tooth in cementum and dentine since no overlying enamel is present. It should be managed by dietary advice and plaque control. When a cavity has formed, the carious dentine should be removed with a round bur (ISO size 012) in the low-speed handpiece; the margins should be cleared first before carious dentine is removed from the part nearest the pulp. The margins should finish at a butt joint without any bevel being created. It is usual to restore these cavities with glass ionomer cement. In some patients who wear dentures, these cavities may extend round three sides of the tooth. Rather than create one large cavity which is then a problem to fill, it is considerably easier to prepare it and fill it in sections. For example, in the case of a lone standing lower premolar, caries affecting the root face of the approximal surfaces should be treated before the caries on the lingual surface in-between is treated, either later in the same appointment or on a different occasion.

8.4 Approximal cavity

SMALL APPROXIMAL LESION

Let us consider a small approximal cavity on the distal surface of an upper premolar. It is not visible by clinical examination and caries affecting dentine is only just observable on a bitewing radiograph. The patient has a high prevalence of caries for his age. Management should consist of:

1 dietary advice,
2 preparation of a very minimal cavity to conserve tooth substance.

An *internal preparation*, sometimes called a tunnel preparation, will be prepared. This was first reported by Hunt (1984).

The first stage of cavity preparation is to gain access to the carious dentine through the fossa at the inner aspect of the marginal ridge. A small round bur in the turbine handpiece is used to make a small cavity just into dentine. The cavity is then dried and examined for the presence of carious dentine. If none is present, the operator should decide on the angle of penetration so that he aims for the carious dentine rather than deviates to one side or towards the pulp. Sound dentine is then removed as the bur is aimed towards the carious dentine. On entering the carious dentine, resistance to penetration will be lost. However, if the operator fails to find the caries, he should stop and redry the cavity to reassess the direction to be taken. When carious dentine has been found then he should proceed to remove it with a round bur (ISO size 012) in a low-speed handpiece using waterspray, moving the tip of the bur in a circular sweep down one side, along the floor and up the other; this is repeated until the resistance of hard dentine is felt. The cavity should then be dried and inspected. Any remaining carious dentine may appear darker in colour than sound dentine; it will also be soft to light pressure from a dental probe; the cavity may be stained with 1% Acid Red in propanol to show where there is remaining infected dentine. All the carious dentine should be removed. No attempt is made to break through the enamel on the approximal surface, nor is any effort made to undermine the marginal ridge — except to remove carious dentine. The intention is to leave all the sound approximal enamel and the marginal ridge intact. The occlusal access cavity is made no larger than is necessary to remove the caries, and as the restorative material is susceptible to abrasion, the smaller the amount exposed occlusally, the better. The margins of the occlusal cavity are smoothed with a chisel. The finished cavity has two holes; the larger is the access orifice and the smaller is the point of penetration of the carious lesion on the approximal surface. Hunt (1984), in a small short-term clinical trial, did not find that any marginal ridge broke away.

This type of cavity is difficult to prepare, particularly for a novice. It is only possible in a carious tooth and cannot be practised in a sound tooth in a manikin.

It is intended that this cavity should be restored with glass ionomer cement (page 139).

LARGE APPROXIMAL LESION

A carious lesion on the distal wall of a lower second premolar with cavitation of the enamel and bacterial penetration of dentine will be considered. On clinical examination, a slight darkening is visible through the intact marginal ridge (Fig. 8.12), and radiographically there is evidence of dentine involvement (Fig. 8.13).

The first stage of cavity preparation is gaining access to the carious dentine to assess its extent. This may be done with a small, round, pear-shaped or fissure bur in the turbine handpiece. The inner aspect of the marginal ridge is drilled away progressively until the dentine is reached, when the bur suddenly drops into the carious dentine as all resistance to penetration disappears (Fig. 8.14). At this stage the bucco-lingual width of the cavity should be approximately 2 mm while the mesio-distal width should be hardly wider than the width of the bur.

The cavity should be dried and examined for caries at the amelo-dentinal junction. If access has been made in the correct place, caries should be present at the junction round the entire cavity. However, sometimes it may be found that the access cavity is placed too far lingually; therefore, in enlarging the cavity, no further extension should occur on this side. By enlarging the cavity until a sound amelo-dentinal junction is found buccally and lingually, the width of the completed approximal part of the cavity on the occlusal surface can be deter-

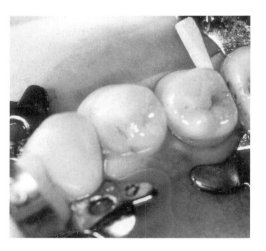

Fig. 8.12 Distal caries in a lower second premolar. A shadow is visible through the marginal ridge.

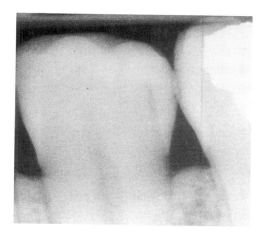

Fig. 8.13 Part of a bitewing radiograph showing distal caries in the lower second premolar.

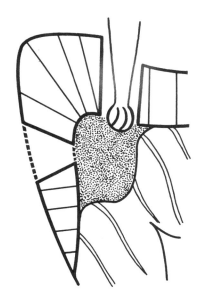

Fig. 8.14 Diagram of approximal caries showing the bur penetrating through the marginal ridge into carious dentine (longitudinal section).

mined. Carious dentine will still remain on the distal amelo-dentinal junction.

Frequently the caries in the dentine has extended to undermine the enamel at the base of the occlusal fissure, causing the fissure to be involved in the outline of the cavity. Extension of the cavity to include the fissure is usually carried out because the fissure may be carious, an occlusal restoration may exist, finishing the margin of the restoration against a fissure could be a potential site for recurrent caries and the extension may contribute substantially to retention of the restoration.

The occlusal extension of the restoration into the fissure system prevents the restoration being displaced approximally. The outline of the occlusal part of the cavity conforms to the general shape of an occlusal cavity by following the fissure pattern. This results in the cavity being narrowest between the cusps and slightly wider than this at the end away from the approximal part, while it is widest at its approximal part.

The preparation of the occlusal part, which is often referred to as a lock or keyway, is straightforward and may be undertaken before completion of the approximal part, the box. Preparation of the keyway is the same as for a simple occlusal cavity and therefore a description will not be repeated. The cavity width should be kept as narrow as possible because unnecessary widening weakens the remaining tooth. The base of the keyway should be just into dentine, and not any deeper except where the dentine is carious.

After the occlusal part of the cavity has been completed, attention is refocused on the approximal caries (Fig. 8.15). It helps to remember that the initial enamel lesion was sited under the plaque which was almost invariably between the approximal contact and the gingival margin, and in line with the contact bucco-lingually. This part of the cavity outline is almost always determined by the extent of dentinal caries and is made no wider than removal of caries dictates. The cavity is extended by following the caries along the amelo-dentinal junction on the approximal surface using a round bur (ISO size 012) in the low-speed handpiece. Although this extension could be done with the turbine handpiece, it is often safer to use the low-speed handpiece as the operator has greater tactile sense and tooth removal is less rapid. Further, the relatively longer bur improves access and the slower rotational speed of the bur reduces the chance of overheating the tooth; waterspray should be used nevertheless. The bur should be taken gingivally gradually to allow adequate cooling. It is moved in a circular motion, down one side, along the gingival wall and up the other side. By keeping the bur on the amelo-dentinal junction, un-

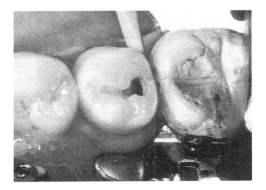

Fig. 8.15 The occlusal part of the cavity has been prepared following the fissure system and carious dentine is present distally.

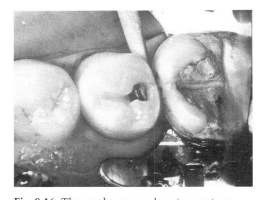

Fig. 8.16 The partly prepared cavity; carious dentine has been removed from the amelo-dentinal junction distally; and the distal enamel wall still remains.

necessary removal of sound dentine should be prevented and the enamel marginal ridge together with much of the approximal surface should remain intact; this prevents damage to both the gingival papilla and the adjacent tooth. Some operators prefer to place a matrix band around the adjacent tooth to protect it from inadvertent damage which can readily occur, particularly when the turbine handpiece is used.

When it is considered that all the marginal caries has been removed, the cavity should be dried and stained with 1% Acid Red in propanol to check for absence of caries at the amelo-dentinal junction (Fig. 8.16). If caries remains at the amelo-dentinal junction on any wall, that part should be extended until the junction is free from caries. The unsupported enamel may then be broken out by the insertion and twisting of a binangled chisel.

Sharp hatchet chisels or gingival margin trimmers should be used to plane the enamel margins of the lingual and buccal walls in an occlusal to gingival direction; these chisels will remove unsupported enamel prisms and create a strong wall with a smooth edge. In cross-section, the wall should meet the external surface of the tooth at right angles to a tangent; this gives a strong margin to the restoration (Fig. 8.17). The outline of the cavity on the approximal surface has rounded corners, and there is no value in squaring it up. When upper premolars are viewed from the palatal aspect, the edge of the palatal wall is usually readily visible; however, this is less common with the lingual wall of a lower premolar. The position of the buccal wall is dependent on the extent of caries and may not necessarily be visible from the buccal aspect; its site has worried operators for many years and it used to be considered necessary to allow access to the margin by a probe tip or toothbrush bristles. However, since the presence of plaque at this margin is not often associated with recurrent caries, a more conserva-

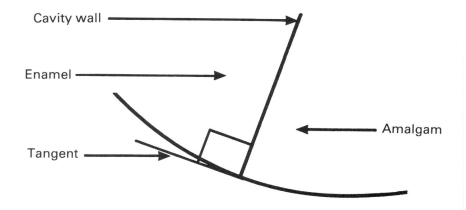

Cavity wall

Enamel

Amalgam

Tangent

Fig. 8.17 The cavity wall should meet the external surface of the tooth at right angles to a tangent (diagrammatic cross-section).

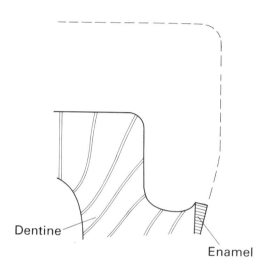

Dentine

Enamel

Fig. 8.18 Cross-section through the gingival wall of the cavity; this aids retention by being concave.

tive cavity is now preferred because the tooth is weakened less. A drawback of a more conservative cavity which has the margin obscured by the adjacent tooth is that subsequent inspection of the margin is impossible. It is preferable if the buccal and lingual walls of the approximal part of the cavity converge occlusally by a few degrees to provide retention. If the convergence is done to excess, the operator will restrict his access and may leave caries at the amelo-dentinal junction under the remaining marginal ridge.

The enamel margin on the gingival wall must be planed with a gingival margin trimmer in a buccal to lingual direction and also from lingual to buccal with the other end of the trimmer. This planing will remove spicules of enamel and unsupported prisms on the wall. Further, the intention is to produce a slight gingival bevel conforming to the prism direction; this is difficult to achieve in practice. The gingival margin of the cavity should be sited where removal of caries dictates; it is preferable if this is supragingival as less gingival irritation is caused by plaque accumulation at the margin. It should not be extended under the gingival papilla unless dictated by the need to remove caries. The use of a round bur to prepare the gingival wall of the cavity often leaves it concave, but this shape aids retention (Fig 8.18).

By preparing the cavity with round burs in the low-speed handpiece, it should be very retentive and not overextended. There should be no need to place additional retentive grooves. However, if the operator is replacing a restoration where the previous cavity had been given an angular shape it may be valuable to place shallow grooves in the dentine of the buccal and lingual walls with a small round bur (ISO size 008) in the low-speed handpiece (Fig. 8.19). The grooves should be more pronounced occlusally. They must neither be placed in enamel nor at the amelo-dentinal junction as unsupported enamel would be created and therefore retention would not be achieved.

By this stage, caries should only remain on the axial wall. It is best removed with a round bur (ISO size 012) in the low-speed handpiece. Only softened dentine stained by the Acid Red dye is removed to avoid damage to the pulp. With extensive caries, a trace of softened dentine not stained by the Acid Red dye may be left on the axial wall but the gingival wall must be free from caries.

The axio-pulpal line angle should be rounded to reduce stress in the subsequent restoration and to prevent the restoration fracturing between the occlusal and proximal parts. The completed preparation is shown in Fig. 8.20.

Many operators fallaciously believe that widening the keyway reduces the chance of fracture of the restoration. They overlook two aspects of mechanics: strength is related to the square of the depth of

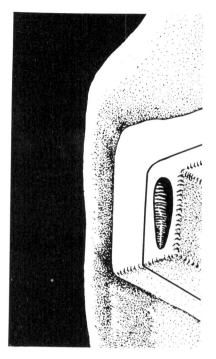

Fig. 8.19 In angular cavities a retentive groove which should be more pronounced oclusally may be placed in dentine on the opposing walls of the box.

the keyway; and rounding the axio-pulpal line angle substantially reduces stress concentration, and hence reduces fracture in a brittle solid such as amalgam. It is rare that extra depth to the occlusal part of the cavity is required, but frequently the operator inadvertently prepares a shallow cavity by failing to reach dentine and also leaves a sharp axio-pulpal line angle; a compromised restoration inevitably follows.

MODIFIED CAVITY

There has been a trend in recent years to prepare more conservative cavities and, in so doing, some operators have failed to produce better restorations because retention has been inadequate or incorrect. The most common conservative cavity is to prepare an approximal box without an occlusal keyway. This is a perfectly satisfactory preparation where a small lesion is treated because the buccal and lingual walls have little flare, enabling effective retentive grooves to be placed in the dentine of the buccal and lingual walls during the process of caries removal. However, where caries has been more extensive the walls will possess greater flare, making such grooves ineffective; an occlusal lock is then necessary. The occlusal lock should make use of the natural contour of the fissure system; the operator must not cut a lock elsewhere, otherwise the cusps are bound to be weakened considerably and the margin angle of the restoration unfavourable.

Where a small carious lesion on the approximal surface of a lower first premolar is being treated, no attempt should be made to extend the cavity across the transverse ridge; instead, reliance for retention should be placed on the grooves in the buccal and lingual walls. With more extensive caries, the cavity must be extended across the transverse ridge to gain adequate retention. The operator should incline the bur perpendicular to the occlusal surface when preparing the keyway and not in line with the long axis of the root. This will prevent excessive weakening of the lingual cusp and unnecessary damage to the pulp (Fig. 8.21).

When caries has affected the root surface approximally, for example gingival to an existing occluso-approximal restoration as a result of food packing from a poor approximal contact, removal of the carious dentine may cause the operator difficulty. First the existing restoration, which is normally amalgam, should be removed with a diamond bur in the turbine handpiece (page 116). This should reveal the carious dentine on the gingival wall of the cavity, which should be removed with a round bur (ISO size 012) in the low-speed handpiece in a similar manner to caries removal for a more superficial approximal lesion

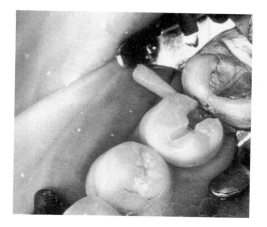

Fig. 8.20 The completed cavity involving the distal surface of the second premolar.

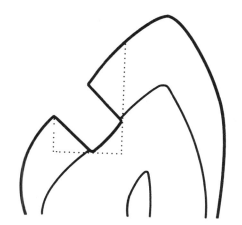

Fig. 8.21 The keyway on a lower first premolar should be perpendicular to the sloping occlusal surface (*solid line*) rather than perpendicular to the long axis of the root (*dotted line*).

(page 101). As the cavity gets deeper, it becomes more important that the operator places the bur in the correct position, i.e. along the gingival margin, and does not allow the bur to wander towards the pulp or towards the gingivae which may not have been protected by a wooden wedge and rubber dam. Inflamed gingivae readily bleed and blood obscures the field of vision. When all the caries has been removed from the margins, which should be planed with a gingival margin trimmer, caries on the pulpal wall may then be removed. The cavity is likely to be retentive since it will be slightly wider just within the margins than at the margin. No intention is made to square up the margins and lose the retentive shape. The cavity is frequently asymmetrical and it is appropriate to leave it in this state; enlargement to create symmetry only weakens the tooth further.

If the approximal root caries is accessible from the buccal or lingual aspect, and there is no existing approximal restoration, the lesion should be treated as a single surface cervical cavity rather than needlessly destroy sound enamel and dentine occlusal to the lesion.

MESIO-OCCLUSO-DISTAL (MOD) CAVITY

Where extensive caries occurs on both mesial and distal surfaces of a molar or premolar (except a lower first premolar), it is usual and almost inevitable that one cavity is prepared embracing both lesions. With an upper first molar, it may be possible to prepare separate mesial and distal cavities leaving the oblique ridge intact. A MOD cavity weakens the cusps more than any other but its damaging effects can be minimized by removing as little sound enamel and dentine as possible. The method of preparation is similar to that for a cavity involving a single approximal surface and does not need to be repeated.

In a molar tooth where there is caries involving one approximal surface and a satisfactory restoration (both clinically and radiographically) in the other approximal surface, the existing restoration is not removed. The extreme part of its occlusal extension may need to be cut away to provide retention and resistance to displacement of the new restoration in the other approximal surface. In doing this the retention of the existing restoration must not be destroyed. The smaller bulk of a premolar tooth makes this technique more difficult and less appropriate so it is usual to create one restoration involving both approximal surfaces.

8.5 Extensive cavities involving cusps

An example will be considered where the disto-lingual cusp has fractured off a restored lower first molar which had a large mesio-occlusal

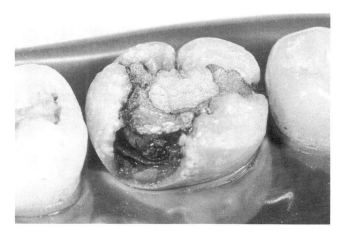

Fig. 8.22 The disto-lingual cusp has fractured off a lower first molar which has an unsatisfactory mesio-occlusal restoration. Carious dentine is present at the exposed gingival margin.

restoration, and there is evidence of caries at the exposed amelo-dentinal junction lingually as well as caries mesially (Fig. 8.22). The operator should remove the unsatisfactory existing restoration with a bur in the turbine handpiece whilst retaining the adequate part of the lining; carious dentine at the affected amelo-dentinal junctions should be taken away with a round bur (ISO size 012) in the low-speed handpiece. Because the distal enamel wall in this example has been undermined by caries, it must be removed to prevent its subsequent fracture. All the cavity margins should be cleared of caries before attention is directed to any remaining on the axial wall. The gingival margin of the lingual aspect of the cavity should be trimmed with a gingival margin trimmer in a similar way to an approximal gingival margin. For preference, the gingival margin should be placed supragingivally but the extent of cusp fracture or presence of caries will dictate its actual position. Distally and lingually the margin may be at different levels; this is quite acceptable and no attempt should be made to create the entire margin at a single level. The lingual wall of the cavity, particularly in its occlusal half, should be in the long axis of the tooth. If it is not, it should be altered with a fissure bur in the turbine handpiece; this is to allow the amalgam to have a good margin angle and sufficient bulk occlusally so that it does not chip subsequently. The cavity wall is then planed with a binangled chisel to remove unsupported prisms. Finally, the carious dentine on the axial wall as indicated by the use of Acid Red dye should be removed, but sound dentine and existing lining cement unassociated with caries

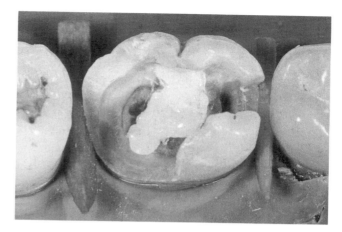

Fig. 8.23 The restoration and caries have been removed from the lower molar; existing lining cement in the centre unassociated with caries has been left.

should be left. The gingival wall of the cavity should be at approximately right angles to the long axis of the tooth, or inclined inwards, to provide some resistance to displacing forces. The prepared cavity is shown in Fig. 8.23. This type of cavity has insufficient retention, so one or more pins are usually used to complement existing retentive features.

The essence of pin retention is a corrosion-resistant pin which is partially inserted into dentine while the remainder of it is surrounded by the restorative material, in this case amalgam. Where a large amount of tooth is missing, a general principle is to place one pin for each missing cusp, or two where the lingual or buccal wall has been lost. As with so many aspects of dentistry, over-use of pins is undesirable because the placing of pin-holes can cause damage.

A pin-hole must not be placed in enamel or at the amelo-dentinal junction because enamel would shatter as it is brittle. Pin-holes are placed in dentine and should be 2.0–2.5 mm deep; their diameter may be 0.5–0.7 mm, according to the manufacturer and type of pin. When the operator prepares these holes, he must take care to ensure that the drill does not enter the pulp, encroach on the amelo-dentinal junction or penetrate the external surface of the tooth. Therefore, only a limited area of dentine is available: a thin strip just within the amelo-dentinal junction. In multirooted teeth, extra care needs to be taken to avoid the furcation.

For the cavity under consideration, one pin placed disto-lingually should be enough to achieve adequate retention since it is being sup-

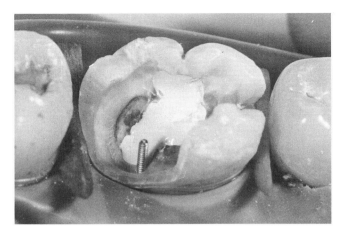

Fig. 8.24 A self-tapping threaded pin has been placed disto-lingually in dentine to provide retention for the restoration.

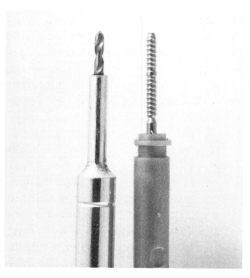

Fig. 8.25 A twist drill (*left*) matched to the size of the self-tapping theaded pin (*right*) for insertion into dentine.

plemented by the form of the remaining cavity (Fig. 8.24). The use of further pins in this example is unnecessary and may court disaster. It is usually easiest for the operator if the long axis of the drill is approximately in line with that of the tooth; variations from this increase the risk of perforation. Where the tooth is tilted, an indication of the long axis may be gained by examining the radiograph and by passing a probe into the gingival sulcus to locate the root surface. The theoretical advantage of a pin and a wall being at different angles is often overridden by the hazards of placing a pin at an angle, as well as the difficulty of angling the handpiece, particularly at the back of the mouth; furthermore, self-tapping threaded pins, which are widely used, are highly retentive when correctly used.

A variety of pin retention systems are produced by a number of manufacturers. It is now standard for the manufacturer to supply pins with matching twist drills (Fig. 8.25). All pin holes are prepared with a slowly rotating twist drill in the low-speed handpiece. The twist drills have a limited life and should be discarded when they become blunt to prevent overheating the tooth and preparing an oversize hole. Many are now made with a shoulder to control depth of penetration and it is important that the drill is used to the correct depth otherwise deep pitched screws may not achieve adequate retention.

The most versatile pin is attached to a contra-angled bur shank and is self-tapping in the prepared hole. The pin is taken to the hole and the bur rotated at low speed and high torque; with some air motors it is necessary to use a speed-reducing head to increase the torque, other-

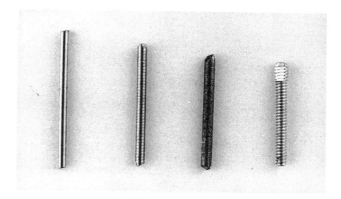

Fig. 8.26 Alternative pin systems. *Left*: a friction-grip pin. *Second from left*: grooved Markley wire (cemented). *Second from right*: sandblasted orthodontic stainless steel wire (cemented). *Right*: self-tapping threaded pin inserted with a spanner.

wise the drill stalls. The pin taps its own thread into dentine and when it can penetrate no further shears at a notch 2–3 mm above the dentine surface. Pins attached to a bur shank are considerably easier and safer to use than older types where the pin was carried to the tooth in a spanner; at the back of the mouth access for the operator's fingers to hold the spanner is also restricted. After insertion the pin should be checked to ensure that it is not loose as a result of faulty technique. If it is, it will need to be removed and cemented into position. Self-tapping pins are considerably more retentive than previous types which were cemented or simply force fitted; and they do not appear to cause clinically significant stresses in the dentine (Fig. 8.26). When pins are placed in teeth with short clinical crowns, it may be necessary to reduce the height of the pin by using a diamond bur in the turbine handpiece to give at least 1 mm coverage with amalgam. In some circumstances it may be possible to bend the head of the pin to keep it within the contour of the restoration, but a special instrument is required so that the dentine is not overstressed.

If the operator inadvertently enters the pulp then root canal treatment may need to be considered, particularly when a crown is planned. An alternative which appears generally successful is to place calcium hydroxide cement in the pin-hole and monitor the condition of the pulp for at least 2 years; in such a case, a crown restoration would be contra-indicated. Should the operator perforate into the periodontium then the cavity margin must be extended to include the defect. With both errors, another hole would need to be placed in a more suitable position to gain retention for the restoration.

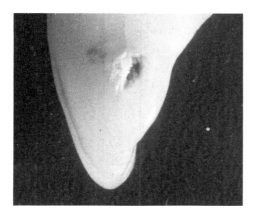

Fig. 8.27 Caries affecting the distal surface of an upper lateral incisor with cavitation of the enamel.

8.6 Cavities in anterior teeth

APPROXIMAL CAVITY

Caries may occur on the approximal surface of any incisor or canine but is far more common on the upper than on the lower teeth. As an example, caries on the distal surface of an upper lateral incisor will be considered. There is cavitation of the surface enamel and bacterial invasion of the dentine (Fig. 8.27).

The first stage is to gain access to the carious dentine and since an adjacent tooth is normally present this is done with a small round tungsten carbide or diamond bur in the turbine handpiece. The bur is used to penetrate through the enamel marginal ridge from the palatal aspect (Fig. 8.28). For preference, the palatal ridge is drilled away as first it is likely that this functional ridge has ceased to be supported by sound dentine, and secondly this approach allows the labial margin of the cavity to be placed where it is almost invisible from the labial aspect. This latter is particularly important as no restorative material, even now, is a perfect colour match under most lighting conditions. The palatal approach does have the disadvantage of giving the operator less direct access. A labial approach is rarely used because it disfigures the face of the tooth. If the adjacent tooth were missing, direct access would be possible.

On reaching the carious dentine, the same round bur is used to extend the enamel walls on the palatal surface of the cavity until the amelo-dentinal junction, palatally, incisally and gingivally, is free from

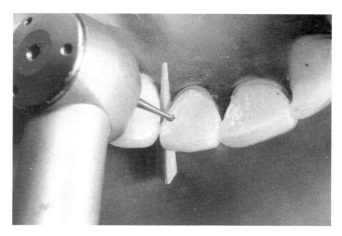

Fig. 8.28 Access being gained through the palatal marginal ridge to the carious lesion.

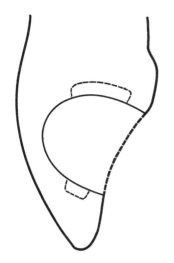

Fig. 8.29 A diagram showing where retentive grooves are placed in dentine.

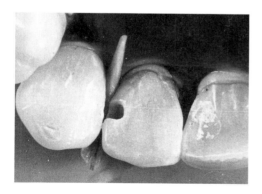

Fig. 8.30 The completed cavity in the upper lateral incisor.

caries. When this is achieved, it is preferable to change to the low-speed handpiece with a medium-sized round bur (ISO size 012). This is used to remove caries from the approximal amelo-dentinal junction working from the palatal towards the labial in a circular motion, along the gingival, up the labial and out incisally. When caries has been removed from the entire amelo-dentinal junction, the outline of the cavity in dentine has been determined. A binangled chisel is then used to remove unsupported prisms from the accessible palatal margins, while a small gingival margin trimmer can be used to remove unsupported prisms on the approximal walls. Where caries has enlarged the cavity further, a watchspring scaler may be used instead to plane the labial and approximal margins. Since the labial enamel wall of the cavity is unlikely to be subjected to severe occlusal pressures, only the most unsupported enamel prisms are removed, leaving much of the weakened enamel plate intact.

The shape of the cavity may offer sufficient retention without the need to place specific retentive grooves. However, when these are used a groove is placed in dentine on the approximal gingival wall, and a short groove, or more often a pit, in the incisal wall. This is achieved with the same bur, or a slightly smaller one (ISO size 010), in the low-speed handpiece (Fig. 8.29). In the larger cavity or in a thin tooth, the incisal wall of the cavity will be virtually little more than the labio-palatal line angle.

The remaining stage is to remove caries from the axial wall and this is aided by the use of dye to stain the infected carious dentine, which can be conveniently removed with a round bur (ISO size 012). The operator should beware of the pulp horn, which is particularly close in the tooth of a young patient. Where the pulp is considered to be in danger, stained carious dentine on the axial wall may be removed with an excavator.

The cavity should be dried and examined from various aspects before proceeding to place the restoration. The shape of the cavity should be similar to Fig. 8.30.

One authority in the past proposed a dovetail shaping of the palatal surface to increase retention. Such extension is unnecessary, particularly with modern materials, and leads to needless removal of enamel and dentine; it results in considerable weakening of the incisal angle. Inverted cone and fissure burs should not be used to prepare this type of cavity because they invariably make the internal aspects of the cavity too angular and threaten the pulp.

The carious lesion is only approached from the labial aspect when the adjacent tooth overlaps preventing a palatal approach or a previous restoration which had a labial approach is being replaced. The outline of the labial part of such a cavity should be kept as small as possible, provided that the approximal part of the cavity can be prepared. The labial opening is not made as large as the equivalent opening for the palatal approach because with direct access the bur can be inserted more from the side of the tooth than from the front.

Extension of the margins of these cavities beyond the carious lesion has been recommended in the past. Such extension leads to unnecessary removal of tooth substance and gingivally can take the margin needlessly close to the gingival tissues, probably causing permanent damage to the gingival papilla. Cavity outline is determined by both caries of enamel and caries of dentine at the amelo-dentinal junction. As all restorative treatment must be combined with the instruction of the patient in the prevention of disease, conservative preparation should be and usually is successful.

Sound enamel and dentine should never be removed needlessly because anterior restorative materials are not as durable and the tooth is weakened. Surveys of the longevity of tooth-coloured restorations report that 50% fail within 5 years. However, it should be realized that these materials can, with correct handling, provide long-lasting restorations.

The cavity which has been described would be suitable for glass ionomer cement and composite resin. Amalgam is now used infre-ever, frequently some modifications are made for two materials: glass ionomer cement   and composite resin. Amalgam is now used infrequently and silicate cement almost never.

In the case of glass ionomer cement, which is adhesive, retentive grooves do not need to be placed on the incisal and gingival walls. But the cavity should still have good resistance form to prevent displacement by occlusal forces.

With composite resins, which do not adhere to tooth substance, marginal leakage and staining may be virtually eliminated by mechanical bonding of the resin into etched enamel. In order to produce a restoration of the correct contour and achieve effective bonding, not only to prevent marginal leakage but also to obtain mechanical retention, it is desirable to apply a small bevel, approximately 0.25–0.5 mm wide, to the enamel margins. The bevel may be readily placed on the palatal margins with a round or pear-shaped bur in the turbine handpiece; if access permits, a fissure bur may be used. However, the placing of a bevel on the approximal margins of a small cavity is impossible because of the proximity of the adjacent tooth. Therefore, in a small cavity retention is also gained by grooves in dentine. Where the cavity is large, there is usually access to enable application of a bevel on all the approximal margins using a small round bur in the turbine handpiece. In the larger cavity, significant retention of the restoration may be required from the etched enamel so the area of bevel must be greater, up to 1 mm wide; when this is done, retentive grooves in dentine can be omitted.

CERVICAL CAVITY

The basic cervical cavity has been covered on page 97 and may be restored with glass ionomer cement or composite resin as well as amalgam. However, the ability of these tooth-coloured materials to bond to the tooth allows alternative cavity preparation.

The V-shaped cervical abrasion may be restored with glass ionomer cement with little or no cavity preparation because of the cement's ability to bond with dentine and enamel. These abrasions are free from caries. Many of these cavities have little or no enamel at the margins, making the acid-etch technique inappropriate.

Where a cervical cavity is completely surrounded by enamel, then it is possible to bevel the margins and use etched enamel for retention of the composite resin restoration. This would eliminate the need to provide retentive grooves. Where the cavity is only bordered by enamel occlusally, retention from etched enamel is limited and would need to be supplemented by one of several ways. Conventionally a groove may be placed in dentine gingivally; second, by using glass ionomer cement in the base of the cavity and overlaying the surface with composite resin (*the sandwich technique*); or third, by the use of an intermediate layer of dentine-bonding agent which adheres to dentine.

ACID-ETCH TECHNIQUE

The technique of using an acid to create pores in the enamel surface for the retention of resin-based restorative materials was first reported in 1955, but a further decade elapsed before the technique was used for fissure sealing in clinical practice, and its use for retaining restorations was not reported until the early 1970s. The delay in applying the technique clinically may be explained by the inability to observe etched enamel until the advent of the scanning electron microscope in the late 1960s. Since then the technique has radically changed the use of resin-based materials. It is remarkable that an effective etching solution had been sitting on the bracket table in dentists' surgeries for almost a century. It is all the more amazing that the creation of suitable pores for retention is best achieved by phosphoric acid, with the optimum concentration being between 30 and 50%. Contrary to one's initial expectations, stronger solutions of acid are less effective

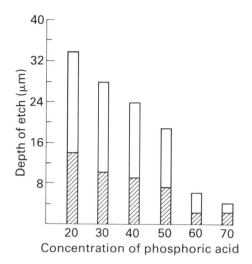

Fig. 8.31 The effect of different concentrations of phosphoric acid on a 1-minute etch of enamel (after Silverstone 1974). □, porous enamel; ▨, enamel removed.

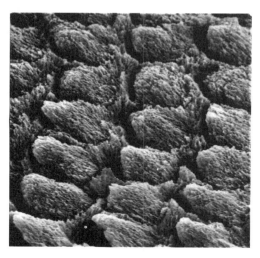

Fig. 8.32 A scanning electron micrograph of sub-surface enamel etched for 1 minute with 37% phosphoric acid; there has been preferential loss of interprismatic mineral (magnification × 1700).

at creating pores; this was clearly shown by Silverstone (1974) and his findings are reproduced in Fig. 8.31. Further, the action of a small drop of phosphoric acid is self-limiting, which is of considerable benefit to the patient. The reason for these unexpected phenomena is the common phosphate ion shared by the acid and enamel. Because calcium phosphate in its various forms is sparingly soluble, the rate of demineralization is controlled. This results in the slow loss of mineral and creation of pores; a typical view of etched enamel is shown in Fig. 8.32. In this illustration, the interprismatic enamel has been preferentially removed, but preferential loss of prism cores may also occur. As is seen from Silverstone's work (Fig. 8.31), a small layer of enamel approximately 10 μm thick is completely removed from the enamel surface while the porous enamel is twice that depth. Silverstone (1975) has reported that the resin penetrates even further than this, approximately 40 μm. The action of the acid is self-limiting because eventually the small volume of solution on the tooth surface becomes saturated with calcium and phosphate ions, so stopping further demineralization. An additional factor is the evaporation of water, concentrating the solution even more.

The most widely used etching solution is 37% orthophosphoric acid and it is usually applied for 1 minute. Silverstone has suggested that a further 1 minute may be needed for some enamel surfaces resistant to etching. However, it would appear possible to achieve adequate etching in 1 minute. Shorter etching times are not advised. The etching solution is supplied in an unbreakable polythene bottle in the same package as the composite resin or unfilled resin. The strength of acid in clinical use depends on the manufacturer and varies from 35 to 50%. More recently it has been supplied as a coloured gel rather than a solution because it evaporates less quickly, is more visible, more controllable and therefore safer.

The mature enamel surface is particularly resistant to etching (Fig. 8.33), probably because of fluoride absorption. For this reason it is advisable to remove the surface layer by applying a bevel to the cavity margin; the bevel may be of variable shape (Fig. 8.34). The resistance of surface enamel is very fortunate for the patient because over-zealous application of acid by the operator will do little harm to the tooth surface. This is possibly part of the reason why etched surface enamel exposed to saliva appears normal after a few days, rather than it being entirely due to the often stated remineralization of enamel.

Etching the sides of prisms is effective in creating pores but does not produce a strong bond when resin is applied, since when the resin is pulled, the bound prisms can come away from the unaffected enamel. For this reason the prisms must be etched on their ends.

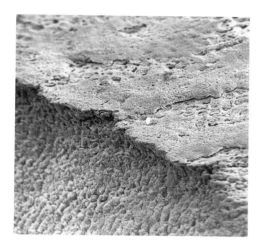

Fig. 8.33 A scanning electron micrograph of a cavity margin showing poorly etched surface enamel (magnification × 500).

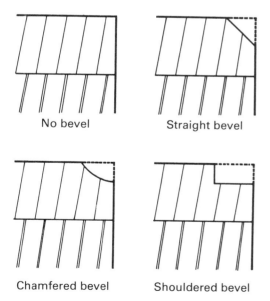

Fig. 8.34 Various forms of cavity margin for composite resin.

Sub-surface enamel etches well and is a good surface for bonding. Effective bonding requires the loose precipitate of various forms of calcium phosphate to be washed off the enamel surface after etching. The surface must be washed with the atomized waterspray for approximately 15 seconds; some authorities have suggested longer but it appears to be to no advantage. Enamel which has been etched but not washed is shown in Fig. 8.35. After washing the tooth is blown with the air syringe to dry the affected enamel, which has a matt chalky appearance. At this stage it is ready for the application of resin. Any contamination of the dried etched enamel by blood, saliva, oil or water will markedly reduce the bond, so it is absolutely *essential* to ensure that the tooth is effectively isolated with rubber dam.

PREPARATIONS INVOLVING THE INCISAL ANGLE

The corner of an incisor may be lost as a result of caries, or it may collapse in the presence of a large approximal restoration, or be broken by traumatic injury. With the latter, the loss of tooth substance is likely to be more horizontal, but the method of restoration is similar whatever the cause, and now relies almost invariably on the retention of composite resin to etched enamel.

The first stage of preparation is the removal of any caries at the amelo-dentinal junction. This is followed by the trimming away of all unsupported enamel prisms. If carious dentine remains on the axial wall, it should be stained with dye and the stained dentine removed with a bur; care must be taken as the pulp horn is likely to be very close.

A bevel at least 1 mm wide should be placed in the enamel round the entire periphery of the cavity, except where it may be impossible gingivally because of the reduced amount of enamel or even its absence. The bevel should penetrate into enamel no more than half its depth; and the operator must take particular care gingivally to keep the bevel in the thin layer of enamel without penetrating into dentine. The bevel is best applied with a round bur in the turbine handpiece; where access is good, a fissure bur may alternatively be used. A round bur will give the bevel thickness, and therefore impart strength to this part of the restoration. The completed preparation is shown in Figs 8.36 & 8.37. As retention is dependent on the area of etched enamel, the bevel should cover a larger area where loss of incisal angle is more extensive. The margin of the restorative material will be at the edge of the bevel, and therefore this cavity margin must be prepared as a smooth continuous line. This calls for a steady hand and is best achieved in one sweep rather than several.

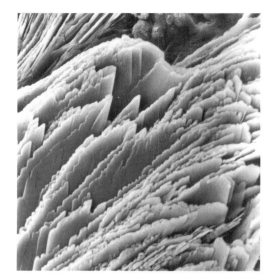

Fig. 8.35 A scanning electron micrograph of sub-surface enamel etched for 1 minute with 37% phosphoric acid which was allowed to evaporate instead of being washed (magnification × 1700). A loose precipatate of salts is present.

A scalloped margin to the preparation has been suggested instead of a continuous smooth margin. Such a margin may appear unsightly if the colour match of the restoration is poor or the restoration subsequently discolours, and it has no mechanical advantage over a continuous smooth margin as retention from etched enamel is so good. Other workers have preferred to use a fine shoulder in enamel instead of a bevel. The choice between the various forms of bevel (Fig. 8.34) would appear to be dictated by operator preference.

The omission of a bevel is unacceptable because surface enamel etches poorly and an overcontoured restoration would be produced. The retention of the restoration is also unlikely to be satisfactory. A bevelled margin is less prone to marginal staining.

Where loss of the incisal angle is very extensive and the operator considers that retention from etched enamel alone would be inadequate, a pin may additionally be placed in dentine, but this is rarely done as there is usually sufficient enamel present.

Some of the older textbooks refer to the placing of retentive grooves and pits in the dentine. This form of retention is now obsolete because of the vastly superior retention from the alternative method of using etched enamel.

8.7 Removal of plastic restorative materials

Restorations may need to be removed because of restoration fracture, caries at the margins, caries elsewhere in the tooth, pulpal problems or discoloration. Regrettably, the operator will spend more time replacing existing unsatisfactory restorations than treating new carious lesions, so a description of their removal is required.

Where an existing restoration must be removed completely, then it should be drilled away by a bur in the turbine handpiece. The operator should remove only the restorative material and neither attempt to enlarge the cavity nor 'freshen up' the margins. The cavity should only be extended where the presence of caries dictates. In some instances the operator can divide up the restoration into small fragments which may be gently elevated by an excavator or chisel; this technique is inappropriate for composite resin retained by etched enamel.

Where only a small part of a large restoration is defective, it is often possible to prepare a small cavity to deal with the defect whilst leaving most of the restoration in place. The operator must ensure that the remaining restoration and the new one will each be retentive. Such a repair is less work than entire replacement and, by virtue of being simpler, errors should occur less often and sound tooth substance should not be sacrificed. Where a pinned restoration is being removed,

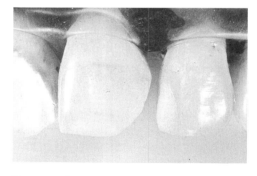

Fig. 8.36 The completed preparation of an upper central incisor for a restoration of the distal incisal angle with composite resin.

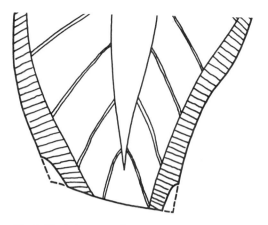

Fig. 8.37 A diagram of a longitudinal cross-section through the preparation involving the incisal angle showing the position of bevels labially and palatally.

the restorative material should be drilled away from around the pins so that they remain for retention of the subsequent restoration.

The drilling out of an amalgam restoration with a bur in the turbine handpiece is easy and benefits from a good volume of water-spray. A diamond bur powders the amalgam more than a tungsten carbide bur, which is liable to project particles of amalgam at the operator and the DSA; for this reason, wearing protective spectacles is essential. Removal of amalgam with a steel bur in a low-speed hand-piece is possible but takes time.

Composite resin may be drilled out with a bur in the turbine handpiece; diamond burs are preferable as the quartz filler in most composite resins soon blunts a tungsten carbide bur, much more quickly than does enamel. Steel burs are quite unsuitable for drilling composite resin apart from the microfilled type as they become blunt within seconds. Since composite resin is tooth coloured, the operator may find it difficult to differentiate it from enamel or dentine. It is necessary to stop and dry the cavity frequently to observe the difference. It is not always essential to remove all the old restoration if part is sound. New composite resin will bond satisfactorily to old.

Glass ionomer cement, unfilled acrylic resin and silicate cement can be drilled away with any type of bur without causing problems for the operator.

Old lining material should not be removed unless caries has spread underneath it, in which case it may be removed with any type of bur.

Bibliography

Elderton R. J. (1984a) Cavo-surface angles, amalgam margin angles and occlusal cavity preparations. *British Dental Journal*, **156**, 319–324.

Elderton R. J. (1984b) New approaches to cavity design. *British Dental Journal*, **157**, 421–427.

Hunt, P. R. (1984) A modified class II cavity preparation for glass ionomer restorative materials. *Quintessence International*, **15**, 1011–1018.

Silverstone L. M. (1974) Fissure sealants: laboratory studies. *Caries Research*, **8**, 2–26.

Silverstone L. M. (1975) The acid etch technique: *in vitro* studies with special reference to the enamel surface and the enamel–resin interface. *Proceedings of International Symposium on the Acid Etch Technique*, pp. 13–39. North Central Publishing Co., St. Paul, Minnesota.

Simonsen R. J. (1980) Preventive resin restorations: three-year results. *Journal of the American Dental Association*, **100**, 535–539.

9 Restoration with plastic restorative materials

The restoring of teeth with amalgam, composite resin and glass iono-mer cement will be described in relation to the cavities prepared in the previous chapter.

9.1 Insertion of amalgam

OCCULUSAL CAVITY

Restoration of the occlusal cavity described in Chapter 8, page 92 will be considered.

The cavity must be absolutely dry for the insertion of the restoration; therefore, the tooth must be isolated effectively, and there is no better way than by using rubber dam; if it were not used for preparation, it certainly should for insertion of the restoration.

The need to place a lining over the dentine has been stressed on page 60 and only a thin layer is required. The technique of using a calcium hydroxide cement will be described. Similar small amounts of the catalyst and base pastes of the cement are dispensed onto a disposable paper mixing pad (Fig. 9.1). These are mixed with a small flat-bladed spatula until the material appears uniform in colour. The tip of a small ball-ended instrument is then dipped in the cement and the material clinging to the tip of the instrument is transferred to the cavity floor, where the cement flows over the dentine. In the occlusal cavity of a lower molar several applications of cement are usually

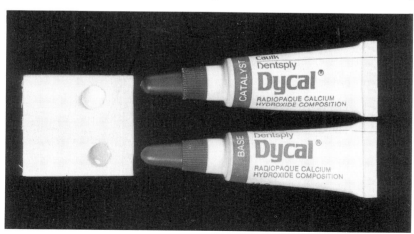

Fig. 9.1 A widely used calcium hydroxide lining cement with similar amounts of each paste dispensed onto the disposable paper mixing pad.

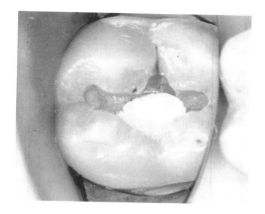

Fig. 9.2 Lining cement has been placed on the cavity floor; this and the walls have been covered with two layers of varnish.

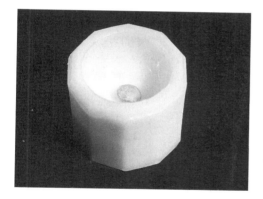

Fig. 9.3 A pellet of mixed amalgam in a small dappen pot.

required to cover the floor of the cavity. The cement sets hard after being on the tooth surface for approximately 1 minute. It is at this stage that any excess cement which flowed onto the enamel must be removed with a sharp excavator. The lined cavity floor will retain the shape of the prepared cavity. There is no need to build up the lining to produce a flat cavity floor as has been suggested by some authorities; such shaping of the lining is of no benefit.

A small pledget of cotton wool should be gripped in a pair of college tweezers and dipped in copalite varnish. This is applied to all the cavity walls and then the cavity is blown dry with the air syringe. The process is repeated and in doing so should have created a thin complete layer of varnish over the lining and cavity walls (Fig. 9.2).

The cavity is now ready for insertion of the amalgam, but first an amalgam plugger which is small enough to fit into all aspects of the cavity must be selected. The amalgam is mixed and placed in a plastic amalgam well or small dappen pot (Fig. 9.3). The nozzle of an amalgam carrier (Fig. 9.4) is pushed into the mass of amalgam and when full is conveyed to the tooth where a small amount of amalgam is dispensed into the cavity. The plugger should then be used to push the amalgam into the base of the cavity and work it into the line angles and retentive features. The use of a cylindrical plugger with a small flat head creates a high packing pressure that is necessary to eliminate porosity and create a strong restoration. When the first increment of amalgam has been thoroughly compressed to form a thin layer over the cavity floor, a further small increment is dispensed from the amalgam carrier. This second layer is then packed into the cavity over a large area to ensure that the thickness of fresh amalgam being compressed is less than 1 mm. If amalgam was packed as a thick layer, only porosity close to· the surface would be eliminated, with voids remaining in the deeper part and union between the increments would be poor. Figure 9.5 shows poor union between increments in the packing of a test specimen when increments were too large and packing pressure was insufficient.

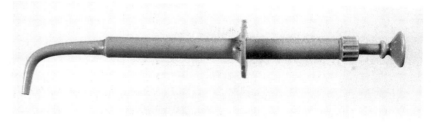

Fig. 9.4 An amalgam carrier manufactured from nylon to minimize clogging.

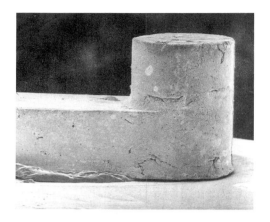

Fig. 9.5 Scanning electron micrograph of a test specimen of packed amalgam showing poor union between increments.

Fig. 9.6 Diagrammatic cross-sections of various marginal finishes that may occur. *Left*: excess amalgam covers the tooth surface. *Middle*: the desired butt joint margin. *Right*: excess amalgam has been carved away creating a step deficiency.

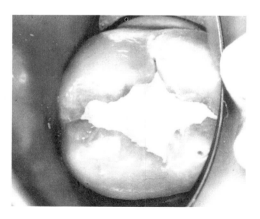

Fig. 9.7 The cavity has been filled with amalgam which has been carved.

Successive layers are inserted and packed until the cavity is overfilled slightly. A pear-shaped burnisher should then be used to give approximate shape to the surface.

As crystallization of the amalgam occurs, its consistency becomes much stiffer and it loses its plasticity; at this stage it is suitable for carving. A sharp-bladed instrument such as a Ward's No. 2 carver or half-size Hollenbach carver should be used to carve away the excess amalgam. To control the degree of carving it is best to work the instrument along the cavity margin. The most convenient way to create the fissure pattern is with a standard excavator, such as the smaller one (Catalogue No. 212/213, Ash Instruments, Dentsply, Weybridge, Surrey) shown in Fig. 4.20 (page 47); an excavator with a large blade should not be used as it produces incorrect contour and margin angles of amalgam which are too acute. The carving instrument may also be moved from enamel to amalgam but considerable care should be taken in using it from amalgam to enamel to prevent too much amalgam being removed and a step deficiency being created (Fig. 9.6).

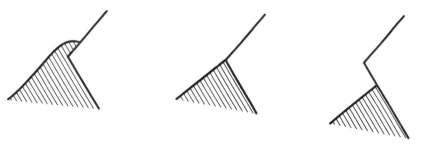

The operator should create what he regards as the correct anatomical form for the tooth, taking into account his previous assessment of the occlusion (Fig. 9.7). When this has been achieved, excess amalgam on the rubber dam around the tooth should be sucked away with the aspirator. The rubber dam clamp is then removed together with the rubber dam. It is now possible to check the occlusion (the principles are detailed in Chapter 16, page 257). The patient should be asked to close the teeth together gently into intercuspal occlusion and hold them in position without pressure. Such an instruction to the patient should be phrased, 'I should like you to close your back teeth together *very gently* and when you feel a contact, hold the teeth in that position *without any force* so that I can see how they meet'.

The degree of separation of the teeth should be noted; this indicates the *size* of the prematurity. When the patient opens his mouth a shiny burnish spot is often seen on the amalgam surface, indicating the *site* of the prematurity. Knowing the size and site of the contact, the operator can now make the appropriate adjustment. It is rare that the occlusal contour is formed correctly before the occlusion is checked, so adjustment is usually necessary. If the shiny burnish mark is not readily visible, the operator may use thin articulating paper to locate the point of contact. When the prematurity has been adjusted, the occlusion should be re-examined to assess whether the contact has been completely corrected or another part of the occlusal surface of the amalgam has come into premature contact. Adjustments should be made until there is no prematurity in intercuspal occlusion. The patient is usually able to confirm that the occlusion 'now feels right' and that teeth on both sides of the mouth meet together evenly. Lateral and protrusive movements of the mandible should be checked to ensure that there is no interference of the restoration in these movements; any prematurities should be eliminated. The larger the restoration, the greater is the potential for interfering occlusal contacts. If there is a prematurity which the operator cannot observe on the restoration, he should check that a piece of excess amalgam is not lying on the occlusal surface of another tooth.

After the restoration has been completely carved and the occlusion corrected, it is desirable to make the surface as smooth as possible to facilitate subsequent polishing. Some operators use a small pledget of cotton wool in a pair of college tweezers; it may be used dry or soaked in methylated spirit; the former is more abrasive. A pear-shaped burnisher may be worked over the carved surface to smooth, and eliminate porosity in, the surface layer. In the past there has been some concern about burnishing at this stage but harmful effects should not occur with amalgam which has been mixed mechanically without excess mercury. The exposed surfaces of the restoration cannot be polished until the amalgam has hardened completely and as that takes some hours polishing is carried out at a subsequent visit. The carved restoration is shown in Fig. 9.8. The patient should be sent away with advice to avoid eating on the anaesthetized side of the mouth; otherwise the soft tissues could be bitten unknowingly. Once the effects of the local anaesthetic have worn off, eating very hard foods should be avoided for the rest of the day. Polishing of the restoration is considered on page 127.

CERVICAL CAVITY

The method of restoring a cervical cavity is similar to that for an occlusal cavity. Although the restoration may not be exposed to occlusal forces, it is still essential that the amalgam is thoroughly packed

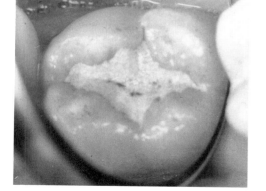

Fig. 9.8 Following removal of the rubber dam, the occlusion has been checked and the shape of the amalgam adjusted.

into the retentive grooves, otherwise its life will be short. Carving in the early stages may be done with a probe, otherwise a Ward's or Hollenbach carver is used.

The operator should aim to reproduce the correct anatomical form of the cervical surface; this requires care with the use of a convex-bladed carver (such as Ward's or Hollenbach) by carving the occlusal and gingival margins separately to avoid a concave surface to the restoration. Whilst the operator should aim for perfection, it is more acceptable to end up with a slightly concave-surfaced restoration than with one which is overcontoured gingivally as this latter will accumulate plaque and encourage gingivitis. Occlusal contacts rarely affect this type of restoration; however, they should be checked.

APPROXIMAL CAVITY

Whereas insertion of amalgam in an occlusal cavity is relatively straightforward, it is more complicated in an approximal cavity because a wall of the tooth is missing and it is necessary to recreate the approximal contour and achieve a contact with the adjacent tooth. The cavity described on page 100 will be restored.

Effective isolation of the tooth is very important and when rubber dam is being used both the tooth being restored and at least the adjacent one must be isolated; the isolation of more teeth in the quadrant usually increases access.

Most of the dentine on the pulpal floor and axial wall should be covered with lining cement. In addition, the inner aspect of the gingival wall should also be lined, leaving 1 mm clear at the margin (Fig. 9.9).

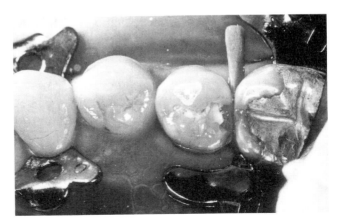

Fig. 9.9 Lining cement placed on the axial and pulpal walls and the inner part of the gingival wall in a disto-occlusal cavity.

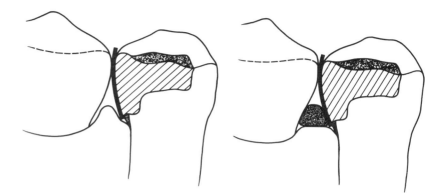

Fig. 9.10 *Left*: the matrix band should extend from just beyond the gingival margin of the cavity to just beyond the marginal ridge. *Right*: the band is held firmly against the tooth by a hardwood wedge.

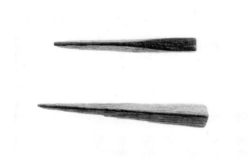

Fig. 9.11 Two commercial tapered hardwood wedges.

Copalite varnish should be applied to give two coats over the lining and every wall of the cavity.

The missing cavity wall is replaced by a matrix band which is usually a thin sheet of stainless steel (35 μm thick) adapted round the tooth. Stainless steel is used because of its strength in thin section and resistance to corrosion or attack by mercury. The width of the band must be sufficient to extend from 0.5 mm apically beyond the gingival wall to 0.5 mm coronally beyond the level of the marginal ridge (Fig. 9.10). The band is normally held in place by some form of commercial holder and kept tight against the tooth at the gingival margin by inserting a hardwood wedge between the teeth (Figs 9.10 & 9.11). There are two main groups of matrix holder: those where the band passes through only one approximal area and those where the band encircles the tooth. In both groups, some commercial band holders are available where the holder and band may be readily dismantled after use to facilitate removal, e.g. Ivory, Tofflemire and Meba. However, with some in the group which encircle the tooth, this is impossible in the mouth unless the band is cut, although they can be taken to pieces out of the mouth for cleaning and band replacement, e.g. Siqveland. A selection of matrix bands is illustrated in Fig. 9.12.

A matrix band, such as the Ivory No. 1, is very useful for replacing the wall of a cavity involving one approximal surface. A very thin band should always be used to give the best adaptation to the tooth surface. Its height from gingival edge to marginal ridge should be just sufficient because excess height will cause damage to the gingival tissues and restrict access for insertion of amalgam. The holder should engage the appropriate holes in the band so that when it is in position it can be drawn close around the tooth. The band is inserted from the occlusal surface, and the gingival edge should be seen to pass over the gingival margin of the preparation just into the gingival sulcus. The holder is

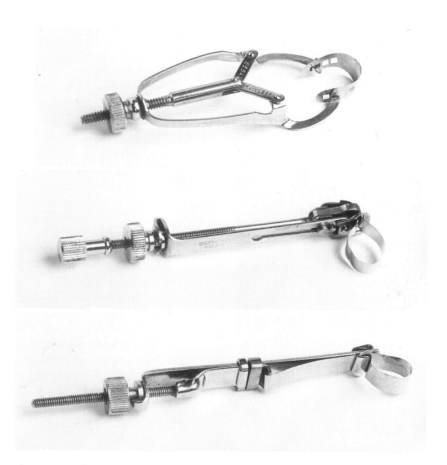

Fig. 9.12 A selection of commercial matrix band holders. *Top*: Ivory No. 1. *Middle*: Meba (Ivory No. 8). *Bottom*: Siqveland.

then partially tightened. A hardwood wedge is inserted from either the buccal or palatal, or occasionally from both sides, to wedge between the adjacent tooth and the band at the level of the gingival wall, thus forcing the band against the gingival margin of the cavity (Fig. 9.13). The wedge should not be placed occlusal to the gingival wall of the cavity, otherwise it would cause a concavity in the approximal surface of the band.

It is very important to ensure that the new restoration will form a good contact with the adjacent tooth; therefore, the band must fit against the contact area on the adjacent tooth; if it does not, the holder should be loosened slightly while the wedge is tight in position gingivally. The approximal contact should be about 1 mm below the level of the marginal ridge provided that the teeth are not abnormally positioned. With premolar teeth the contact is little more than a point, whereas with molar teeth it is larger and may be as much as 2–3 mm

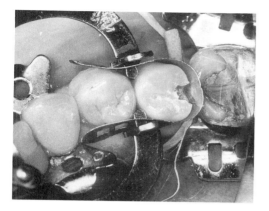

Fig. 9.13 A matrix band is wedged in place to form the cavity wall of the disto-occlusal cavity.

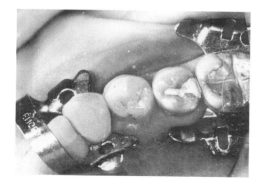

Fig. 9.14 The amalgam restoration has been carved, and the occlusion will be checked for absence of premature contacts after removal of rubber dam.

wide and 1 mm in height. To improve the approximal contour the band may be contoured with a pear-shaped burnisher. The approximal contact prevents drifting of teeth and also food packing, which is both unpleasant for the patient and destructive on the periodontium. If a tooth is restored with a deficient approximal contact, a periodontal pocket may develop within a matter of months as a result of food packing; also, dental caries may subsequently occur on the newly exposed root surface. This carious lesion may miss detection until it is large, and it is also not so easily accessible to burs and excavators during the removal of carious dentine.

When the band is correctly placed it should be impossible to move it away from the gingival wall with an instrument such as a small amalgam plugger. Should it move, the wedging must be improved. A piece of dental floss (approximately 300 mm long) is passed between the contact of the band and adjacent tooth to rest on the wedge; it will be used after insertion of amalgam to remove any gingival excess.

The approximal part of the cavity is filled with amalgam before the occlusal part and it is particularly important to place the amalgam in small increments, working it into the corners and compressing it thoroughly before adding more, because underpacking of a restoration invites early failure. After filling the entire cavity to excess, the amalgam is allowed to commence crystallization before most of the occlusal excess of amalgam is removed with a Ward's or Hollenbach carver. A probe is used to remove excess amalgam from the marginal ridge. The holder is then unscrewed and detached from the band; this is only possible with certain holders. The wedge is taken out and the band slid out by being rotated sideways, thereby avoiding any direct pull occlusally which might damage the marginal ridge. Excess amalgam is then carefully carved away from the approximal surface using a Ward's carver, a Hollenbach carver or a probe, whichever is the most suitable. If a deficiency is found, the restoration must be taken out and replaced. It is particularly important to remove any gingival excess of amalgam early, as it is easy to do while the amalgam is soft; if it were allowed to remain it would provide a site for plaque accumulation with accompanying gingival inflammation. After clearing most of the approximal excess, the piece of dental floss which had been previously inserted may be used to remove small traces of excess at the gingival margin. Care must be taken neither to cut into the restoration nor to damage the approximal contact.

The occlusal surface is carved until it is considered correct (Fig. 9.14) and the rubber dam is then taken off for the occlusion to be checked. It is particularly important that the patient closes his teeth together *very gently* to prevent fracture of the marginal ridge. The procedure of checking occlusal prematurities is similar to that for an occlusal restoration (page 121). If the marginal ridge were to be bitten away by the patient, then it is usually necessary to replace the restoration.

EXTENSIVE CAVITY

Where a large part of the tooth is missing, it may be possible to replace the missing walls of the cavity with a proprietary matrix band which encircles the tooth; alternatively, a customized band must be made. Whichever band is used, it must be wedged interdentally to prevent excess amalgam being packed into the gingival sulcus. However, if the band moves away from the gingival wall on the buccal or lingual aspects of the tooth during packing of amalgam, the gingival excess is readily accessible to carving after the band has been taken off.

Where a proprietary band will not fit, the operator may choose to use a proprietary band without a holder (e.g. Caulk Auto Matrix, from Caulk Co., Dentsply, Weybridge, Surrey), or adapt either a stainless steel orthodontic band or a copper band. These alternative matrix bands are shown in Fig. 9.15. The Caulk Auto Matrix and the orthodontic band are very suitable where the gingival margin of the prepared tooth is at a similar level all the way around the tooth, but they are less appropriate where there is a deep box. With the Caulk Auto Matrix a band of sufficient circumference and height is chosen and placed over the tooth; it is held steady while a special instrument is used to tighten the band. It is wedged approximately before packing of amalgam proceeds in the normal way. With the orthodontic band, one of appropriate size is chosen and placed over the tooth; if the marginal fit is not quite right, the band is removed and the margin adapted with special pliers before retrying the band on the tooth. The band is held in position by being wedged approximately before amalgam is inserted in the normal way. With the copper band, a proprietary matrix band is

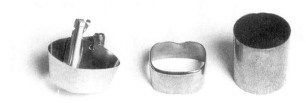

Fig. 9.15 Various bands which may be used for an extensive cavity. *Left*: Caulk Auto Matrix. *Middle*: stainless steel orthodontic band. *Right*: copper band.

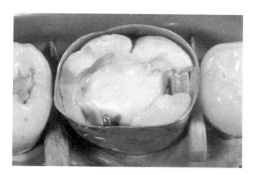

Fig. 9.16 A copper band has been adapted to fit round a lower molar; it is held approximally with wedges.

tried over the tooth first and then a copper band of similar size is chosen. To make the copper more malleable, it is annealed by heating it in a bunsen flame and then it is immediately immersed in a small container of methylated spirit which prevents surface oxidation of the copper.

The softened band should be slipped over the tooth to assess its fit and shape. The band is trimmed with a special pair of metal-cutting scissors so that its gingival contour follows the soft tissue profile; and the rough edges must be smoothed with a carborundum stone prior to insertion in the mouth. Its gingival fit should be reassessed and modified where necessary. The occlusal height of the band should also be adjusted to be at a level just above the marginal ridge to facilitate packing of amalgam. When the band has been completely adjusted it is held in place with wedges interdentally (Fig. 9.16). If it is unstable, additional support may be gained by using composition placed around the outside of the band.

With all large cavities it is very important to ensure that the amalgam is inserted in small increments, each of which is thoroughly packed into the retentive features, around pins where present, and into all the external line angles of the cavity to ensure a strong homogeneous well-fitting restoration. It is tempting to pack the amalgam with a large instrument as the procedure is done more quickly but the restoration will be porous and deficient at the margins; therefore, a small instrument must be used whether or not a spherical amalgam alloy is being used.

Once crystallization has commenced the band may be removed. In the case of a stainless steel orthodontic or copper band, it will need to be cut through on the buccal or lingual aspect with a diamond bur in the turbine handpiece, with care being taken to avoid damage to the underlying tooth or amalgam. The amalgam is carved in a similar way to that described for the approximal lesion but, because the restoration is larger, more care is required to achieve the correct shape and to take account of the occlusion, both intercuspal and functional. If the copper band or orthodontic band had been trimmed out of occlusal contact, it could have been left on the tooth for 24 hours before its removal. This is more common where the amalgam is being used as a core for a crown. It is essential that the band has no sharp edges occlusally to avoid damage to the tongue or cheek.

9.2 Polishing of amalgam

At a subsequent visit, the surface of a set amalgam restoration should be polished to reduce plaque accumulation and corrosion.

The restoration is first examined for correct occlusion, approximal contacts, marginal integrity and contour. If the approximal contact or the integrity of the margins is found to be deficient, it is usually necessary to replace the restoration. Should the occlusal contacts be slightly premature, they should be located with articulating paper if they are not readily visible as shining spots, and adjusted using a finishing bur in the low-speed handpiece. Should the gingival contour have been overbuilt, the excess amalgam must be trimmed away with a flame or tapered finishing bur in the low-speed handpiece. Care must be taken to avoid damage to the tooth around the restoration, the adjacent tooth or the gingivae. To facilitate trimming of the restoration, the gingivae may be effectively isolated and retracted by application of rubber dam. After the restoration has been contoured to shape, something which should have been created at the previous visit, a slightly blunt pear-shaped finishing bur, or even a blunt round steel bur, should be run over the amalgam surface at a speed of aproximately 8000 r.p.m. The intention is not to remove the entire surface layer but to eliminate the roughness left by carving. By keeping the position of the bur on the move, it should be possible to avoid it digging in and causing a rippled surface. Any marginal catches detected by passing a probe across the margins should be eliminated; at the extensions of the fissure a small blunt round bur (ISO size 008) is most suitable. Over-enthusiastic use of the bur can easily destroy a well-carved restoration and result in an undercontoured restoration. Where access to the restoration is particularly good, such as the palatal aspect of an approximal restoration, the amalgam may be smoothed with a tapered finishing bur or a fine sandpaper disc.

After using the finishing bur, an abrasive rubber cup, wheel or point may be used to smooth the more accessible parts of the surface

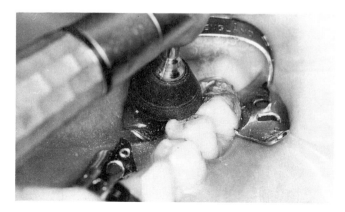

Fig. 9.17 A rubber cup being used to smooth the surface of the amalgam.

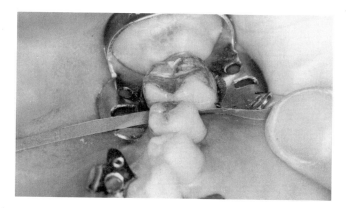

Fig. 9.18 A polymer-based polishing strip being used to polish the amalgam on the approximal surface.

(Fig. 9.17). In any polishing procedure the surface is treated with a range of abrasives which become successively finer.

The gingival margin of an approximal restoration is only likely to be accessible to a polishing strip. These strips, which have a linen or polymer base, are available in a range of widths and grits. The approximal contact should not be abraded during the polishing process and, to allow the strip to pass freely gingival to the contact, the strip must often be cut narrower with a pair of scissors, although manufacturers have now started producing very narrow strips (Fig. 9.18). Initially a coarse strip is used, followed by a fine one.

Completion of polishing is achieved with abrasive slurries. The interdental finishing strip should be coated with a pumice paste, conveniently made by mixing pumice with glycerine or even acidulated fluorophosphate gel. This paste should be worked over the approximal surface with the strip. A very small cup brush should be loaded with the paste and worked over the other surfaces of the restoration. The brush is rotated slowly (3000 r.p.m.) to avoid scattering the paste everywhere, and the position of the brush should be kept on the move to avoid ridges being worn into the surface of the restoration (Fig. 9.19).

The tooth is then washed to remove particles of pumice and dried to check for a smooth surface. If imperfections exist, further pumicing must be done.

Whiting, or alternatively plain zinc oxide, mixed with methylated spirit to a stiff paste is next used on the abrasive strip interproximally, and in a clean dry cup brush on the other surfaces. The speed of rotation should be higher than that used for applying pumice and, as

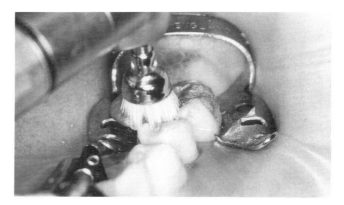

Fig. 9.19 A cup brush with pumice being used to smooth further the surface of the amalgam.

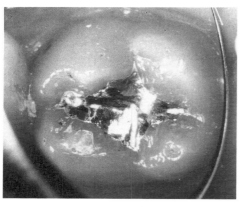

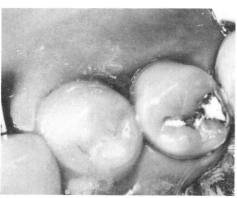

Fig. 9.20 *Top*: The completely polished occlusal restoration. *Bottom*: The completely polished approximal restoration.

the methylated spirit evaporates, the surface will start to shine. The final lustre is best produced with the paste applied in a flexible rubber cup (Young's). The restoration should now have a high gloss without any surface imperfections (Fig. 9.20). If the surface is rippled or scratched, it indicates insufficient pumicing. If the surface is porous, it reveals that the restoration was insufficiently packed and that the restoration should really be replaced, though if it is of a minor nature it may be considered insufficient to justify replacement of the restoration.

All polishing should be done with an intermittent technique to dissipate the heat of polishing. Failure to do so could cause pulpal damage.

If an amalgam restoration is not polished, it will accumulate more plaque on its surface; this may promote gingivitis or recurrent caries. An unpolished restoration is also more prone to corrosion because of its rough surface, and deep destructive pitting corrosion is much more likely to occur.

9.3 Insertion of composite resin

PREVENTIVE RESIN RESTORATION

A lining of a calcium hydroxide cement is placed on the exposed dentine (as described on page 118). In view of the small size of the cavity, it may be easier to apply the lining cement with a periodontal probe rather than a lining applicator because of its smaller diameter. Varnish is neither placed over the lining nor on the cavity walls.

The enamel margins of the cavity and the sides of all the fissures (up to 2 mm from the centre) are etched with phosphoric acid. Etching has been considered in Chapter 8 (page 113), but the clinical procedure is given here. Phosphoric acid gel or liquid is placed in a shallow dappen pot and into this is dipped a brush, pledget of cotton wool or a small piece of sponge held in college tweezers. The acid is applied for 1 minute. After this, the tooth surface is washed for not less than 15 seconds with a waterspray from the 3-in-1 syringe. The tooth is then dried with air from the 3-in-1 syringe for a similar period, following which the etched enamel should have taken on a frosted appearance.

Sealant resin is then placed on the cavity walls and on the etched enamel of the cusp slopes with another brush. Pooling of the resin in the cavity should be avoided and any that does should be removed with a dry brush. The resin is then polymerized with light for 15 seconds before the cavity is filled with posterior composite resin using a flat plastic instrument; the occlusal surface is finished flush with the enamel margins. The surface of the restoration and the fissures are recoated with sealant resin which is then cured for 1 minute. The restoration is then examined to check that there are no deficiencies. If any are present, further sealant would need to be applied and cured.

The rubber dam is then removed so that the occlusion can be checked. If the composite resin has been overbuilt, the offending place will need to be identified with articulating paper and adjusted using an abrasive point in the low-speed handpiece.

The use of a coloured sealant has become increasingly widespread so that the operator can readily see the sealant and, particularly, that it is in place on subsequent occasions. The patient and his parents can also see where the 'prevention' has been carried out, and this can sometimes be very helpful in encouraging patient motivation.

ANTERIOR APPROXIMAL CAVITY

The tooth should be adequately isolated with rubber dam, and the dentine apart from that within 1 mm of the margins should be lined with a calcium hydroxide cement (Fig. 9.21). The technique of lining is the same as that described for amalgam in Section 9.1 (page 118) but copalite varnish is not applied.

It is next necessary to place a matrix strip to form the missing wall of the tooth, and because the restorative material is more fluid than amalgam and some composite resins may become discoloured during removal of a stainless steel band, a different type of matrix strip is used. Frequently these strips are made from cellulose acetate or mylar.

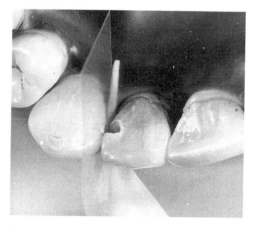

Fig. 9.21 A lining has been placed on the axial wall of the distal cavity in the lateral incisor; and a mylar matrix strip has been wedged in position.

A 20–30 mm length of strip should be taken and slid through the approximal contact from the incisal edge down past the gingival margin of the cavity just into the gingival sulcus, ensuring that it does not trap the gingival papilla or rubber dam. Where the teeth are tight together they may be wedged apart with a wooden wedge to ease the passage of the strip. About 10 mm of the strip should extend onto the palatal side. When the strip is in the correct position it is held tight against the gingival wall of the tooth with a wooden wedge (Fig. 9.21). This wedging is extremely important to prevent gingival excess of restorative material, which is virtually impossible to remove from this position once it has set. The strip should be brought round the tooth to see that it conforms to the shape of the tooth and will give the correct contour, and it should be burnished to give a better contour if necessary. Where it is impossible to achieve a good contour all the way around, the strip should be contoured to give the best possible fit in the parts where subsequent trimming of the set material will be most difficult, i.e. interproximally, therefore placing the greatest excess in the most accessible positions for finishing, i.e. palatally or labially.

After the cavity has been lined with a calcium hydroxide cement, the bevelled enamel at the periphery of the cavity is etched to provide retention for the composite resin. The acid gel is then placed on the enamel margin of the cavity, with the operator being careful to avoid unnecessary acid contamination of the tooth surface away from the cavity; the adjacent tooth will be protected by the matrix strip already in position. The acid should remain on the enamel for 1 minute.

The tooth surface is then washed for 15 seconds with the atomized waterspray from the 3-in-1 syringe; the spray should be collected by the large bore aspirator. The tooth is then dried thoroughly with compressed air from the 3-in-1 syringe to reveal the etched enamel, which has a matt chalky appearance.

The bonding resin should be dispensed onto a paper pad or into a dappen pot. It is picked up with a brush and applied to the cavity margins. If excess pools in the cavity, it should be absorbed by another dry brush. The low viscosity of the resin ensures good contact with the etched enamel. The resin is then polymerized with intense light for 15 seconds.

The composite resin of appropriate shade is then dispensed onto a paper pad. The material is picked up by a flat plastic instrument (preferably a surface-coated one) and transferred to the cavity where it is pushed into the retentive features. For the large cavity it may be necessary to fill it in increments. It is essential to avoid deficiencies. The matrix strip is then brought round the palatal side of the tooth and held in position with a pear-shaped burnisher. As it is adapted,

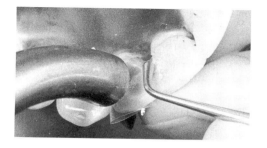

Fig. 9.22 The curing light being applied to the palatal surface of the restoration. The matrix strip is held with an instrument to allow the light to cure the material.

excess material is usually extruded. The light source is applied to the palatal surface by the DSA as the operator is holding the burnisher palatally and the matrix labially against the tooth (Fig. 9.22). The light is switched on for 1 minute before it is moved to cure the labial side for a similar time. After this, the strip may be removed and the restoration examined for deficiencies. If any are found, it may be possible to add material to fill the defect and then recure it, or part of the restoration will need to be removed before material can be introduced into the defect and cured.

TRIMMING

Composite resin is too hard to be carved with sharp hand instruments so it must be trimmed with rotary instruments, preferably in the low-speed handpiece to minimize damage to the enamel which could readily occur with the turbine handpiece. Easily accessible excess may be removed with a 15 mm diameter flexible coarse abrasive disc (such as Soflex, from 3M Health Care, Loughborough, Leicestershire) (Fig. 9.23), particularly on flat surfaces; on the concave palatal surface a small diamond or carborundum point is suitable. In the interproximal and cervical regions, where every effort should have been made to avoid excess, a tapered diamond or tungsten carbide bur in the low-speed handpiece with waterspray is effective. Care must be taken neither to overtrim the restoration causing a deficiency nor to damage the enamel surface. The use of waterspray with stones and burs prevents overheating and clogging, and allows more efficient trimming.

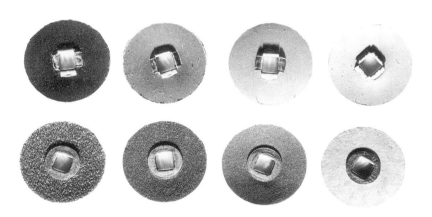

Fig. 9.23 Soflex flexible abrasive discs. *Left to right*: coarse, medium, fine and superfine. *Top line*: rear surfaces progress from dark to light. *Bottom line*: abrasive surfaces progress from coarse to superfine.

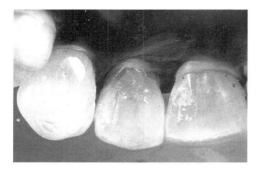

Fig. 9.24 The palatal surface of the finished restoration in the distal surface of the lateral incisor; the restoration does not show from the labial aspect.

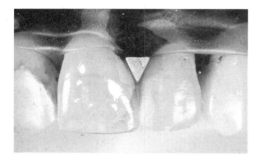

Fig. 9.25 A trimmed crown form tried over the distal incisal angle preparation.

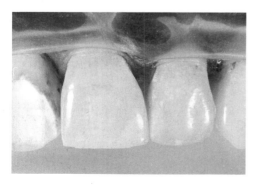

Fig. 9.26 The completed distal incisal angle restoration.

When excess has been removed, the surface of the restoration may be smoothed with specially manufactured fine abrasive flexible discs (Soflex) (Fig. 9.23); these come in a range of abrasivity and are used dry. Progressively finer discs are used, with the finest ones smearing the surface to produce a very smooth finish.

On the approximal surface no further attention should be necessary at the contact or immediately gingival to it because of efficient wedging of the matrix strip, but palatally and labially trimming of slight excess may be required. The most convenient method is to use a flexible abrasive strip. A suitable one is available with a central region free of abrasive to allow it to be slid into position gingival to the contact; at one end is coarse abrasive and at the other fine abrasive. If the strip is too wide, it may be cut narrower with a pair of scissors, as has been described for the finishing of amalgam (page 129).

After trimming, the restoration should be examined to ensure that there is no porosity in the surface layer. Sometimes further material may be added but it may be necessary to replace the restoration if a large void has been exposed. The trimmed restoration is shown in Fig. 9.24.

After removal of the rubber dam the occlusion should be checked and any necessary adjustments made following identification of premature contacts with articulating paper, first in intercuspal occlusion and subsequently in functional occlusion. As composite resin is not a water-based material, it does not need to be protected with varnish during the initial period after insertion, as does glass ionomer cement.

RESTORATION OF AN INCISAL ANGLE

The technique for this type of cavity is very similar and differs only in the choice and adaptation of the matrix former.

The use of preformed celluloid crown forms may have attractions for the inexperienced operator, but it is often found that the standardized contour of the crown form is not an entirely appropriate shape for the worn adult tooth being restored. The crown form must be trimmed carefully to shape (Fig. 9.25). Further, the accurate placing and wedging of the gingival margin of a crown form full of composite resin may on occasions be difficult; if the operator is careless there will be a large amount of gingival excess interproximally, from where it is very difficult to remove the set composite resin. To avoid air being trapped at the incisal corner inside the crown form filled with composite resin, the corner should be perforated with the tip of a probe prior to filling. A way of straightening the incisal edge is to crimp the incisal edge of the filled crown form with college tweezers prior to and during setting.

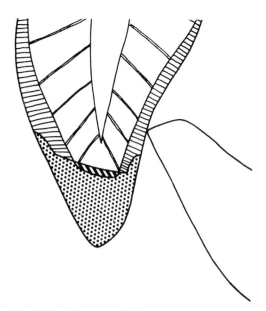

Fig. 9.27 A diagram of a longitudinal cross-section through the incisal angle restoration.

Instead of a crown form, a standard matrix strip which is wedged at the gingival margin may be used. By positioning it carefully as it is brought round the tooth, it is possible to achieve an approximal contact with the adjacent tooth and a good contour of the tooth. It is usual to hold the strip in position on the palatal side with a finger as insertion of composite resin is commenced. When the entire corner has been built up, the labial aspect of the strip is adapted and held with a pear-shaped burnisher while the curing light is applied to the labial surface for 1 minute by the DSA. The burnisher is then moved to the palatal side to hold the strip in position. The DSA then places the curing light against the palatal surface to cure the material from that side for 1 minute. The matrix strip may then be removed to check that there are no deficiencies. There is usually considerable incisal excess, which is fortunately readily accessible to trimming with discs. The completed restoration is shown in Fig. 9.26.

With a restoration involving the incisal edge, it is not only important to examine intercuspal occlusion and remove any premature contacts but also to ensure that none exist in protrusive and lateral mandibular movements (Fig. 9.27).

CERVICAL CAVITY

For a cervical cavity the technique is very similar except that a different type of matrix support is used. A transparent matrix cover should be selected and tried over the cavity. After the composite resin has been inserted in the cavity, the matrix cover is placed over the material to contour it. The cover is held in position and it is important that it rests on tooth all the way around its periphery, otherwise the restoration is very likely to be undercontoured (Fig. 9.28). After the material has set, the matrix cover can be removed and the composite resin trimmed with suitable abrasive discs, stones or burs to remove excess.

Some operators prefer to adapt the composite resin freehand and so do not use a matrix cover, but the freehand technique is more difficult for the inexperienced operator.

RESTORATION OF POSTERIOR TEETH

A number of clinical trials have been carried out into the use of posterior composite resin in the occlusal surfaces of molar and premolar teeth. Five-year results are now available and demonstrate that the material fares as well as amalgam, with over 90% being clinically acceptable and no difference being apparent in wear patterns whether used in large or small cavities, molars or premolars, occlusal or occluso-

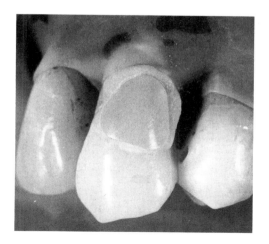

Fig. 9.28 A matrix cover placed over composite resin in a cervical cavity.

approximal cavities. Clinical trials have not reported their use for cuspal restorations, where stress and wear are likely to be more significant.

The type of cavity that has been used has been very similar to that for amalgam, probably because many cavities had amalgam replaced with composite resin for good clinical reasons. Where the operator can prepare a new cavity, emphasis is on keeping it small and using retentive features created by caries removal. There is debate about bevelling the margins. Bevelling the occlusal margins increases the surface area of composite resin which can then be worn away; it is considered unnecessary on cusp slopes, as the angle of cavity preparation will expose prisms end on; no differences with regard to the presence or absence of bevels have been noticed in the success rate of restorations in clinical trials. Theoretically, bevelling provides a better surface for bonding and *in vitro* research has supported the use of bevels.

To ensure that the approximal contact is subsequently tight the interproximal space should be prewedged during cavity preparation. It has the additional advantage of holding the rubber dam in position. To ensure good bonding at the gingival margin it is essential to isolate the tooth with rubber dam. A lining should be placed on the dentine. The enamel margins should be etched for 1 minute, washed for 15 seconds and dried for 15 seconds. Unfilled resin is then applied to the etched enamel with a brush, and then polymerized for 15 seconds with the curing light.

A matrix band is placed, ensuring that it is well wedged gingivally and that it has been burnished against the adjacent tooth to give a good approximal contour. An increment of composite resin is placed into the gingival part of the cavity and adapted with pluggers. This is cured for 1 minute before a further increment is inserted, adapted and cured. An incremental technique reduces the chances of voids, minimizes setting contraction and avoids failure to cure at the base of thick sections, the so-called 'soggy bottom'. After the final increment has been cured, the matrix band and wedge are removed and the restoration checked for voids. Excess composite resin should be in readily accessible places and is best trimmed away with abrasive points and discs in the low-speed handpiece. Minor excess on the approximal surface may be smoothed with finishing strips.

After the rubber dam has been removed, the occlusion must be checked in intercuspal occlusion and in lateral and protrusive mandibular movements. Premature contacts may be detected by articulating paper. The surface of the restoration may be finally smoothed with abrasive rubber cups and points.

Restorations in posterior composite resin are indicated particularly for upper premolars where amalgam restorations would look unsightly. However, it is a difficult material to use well and it is not easy to achieve tight approximal contacts. Its use in extensive cavities involving cusps is still experimental.

9.4 Insertion of glass ionomer cement

When glass ionomer cement is to be used as the restorative material, the prepared cavity must be effectively isolated from contamination by saliva or blood. Where sound dentine has been exposed during cavity preparation, it is considered advisable to place a lining cement as already described for amalgam on page 118, but copalite varnish is not applied because it would reduce the adhesion of the cement to enamel and remaining dentine. The lining is used to protect the pulp from the irritant effects of bacterial penetration as a resultant of an imperfect seal rather than the material's own irritancy. Where an insensitive abrasion cavity is being restored without any mechanical cavity preparation, the enamel surface should be cleaned with the manufacturer's recommended conditioner; in the past this was citric acid but dilute polyacrylic acid is currently advocated. The conditioner is applied for 10 seconds before being washed away with the waterspray and dried with the air from the 3-in-1 syringe. The tooth surface is then ready for the application of glass ionomer cement. Apart from removing plaque and proteinaceous debris, the acid conditioning improves the bonding of the cement to dentine.

An appropriate shade of cement should be chosen by referring to the manufacturer's shade guide. The powder and liquid should each be dispensed in the correct amounts onto a glass slab or a disposable paper mixing pad; this should be done when the operator is ready for the cement to be mixed, not before, to avoid evaporation of water.

The cement is mixed with a spatula either by adding the correct amount of powder to the liquid or by adding increments of powder to the liquid to achieve a putty consistency; the cement should have a smooth texture. The mixed cement should be introduced incrementally and quickly into the cavity, ensuring that all aspects are filled without voids. With an approximal cavity the matrix strip is adapted as for composite resin and held until the cement has set. Then the strip may be peeled back and removed.

The excess material, and there usually is excess, should be carved from the tooth surface, with a sharp excavator or a sharp sickle scaler, whilst it is in a rigid but carveable stage before the material becomes too hard. Care must, of course, be taken not to overcarve or exert too much force on the restoration as part might be dislodged. The restoration must then be coated to protect it from moisture loss or water gain during the early hours of its life. Formerly a layer of varnish was recommended but now a bonding resin which is cured by light is advised. If no protective layer is applied the restoration will have a short life.

The rubber dam can now be removed and the occlusion checked. Any prematurity should be adjusted with a sharp steel bur in the low-speed handpiece and the surface recoated. After insertion the colour of the restoration frequently appears a slight mismatch. However, during the subsequent few hours the setting reaction of the cement continues and the colour match improves as the cement darkens and becomes less opaque.

At the next visit, final smoothing of the restoration may be performed using white stones, tungsten carbide burs and abrasive rubber cups in the low-speed handpiece.

SANDWICH RESTORATION

In the last few years, the sandwich restoration has been promoted. In essence, glass ionomer cement is applied to the base of a cavity and the surface is veneered with composite resin (Fig. 9.29). The purpose is to maximize the adhesion of the cement to the dentine and to take advantage of the superior appearance of composite resin. This type of restoration is often placed in a cervical cavity where there is only enamel on the occlusal cavity margin.

Glass ionomer filling cement is placed in the cavity such that it is filled short of the surface. The cement should be used at a filling consistency and be applied in a thick layer. After the cement has set (not less than 5 minutes), the enamel margin should be etched for 1 minute. During the last 15 seconds, the acid may be allowed to etch the cement. The surface is then washed for 15 seconds and dried thoroughly. The etched surface is coated with bonding resin which is subsequently cured for 15 seconds. The composite resin is then applied, contoured and cured for 1 minute. This technique has been criticized for being complicated, technique-sensitive and prone to failure at the gingival margin. As with so many aspects of operative dentistry, technique is all important. Failures can be attributed to using too thin a mix of glass ionomer cement, too thin a layer of glass ionomer cement, etching the cement too soon and for too long. Some authorities have recommended delaying etching the glass ionomer cement and applying the composite resin to a subsequent appointment in order to minimize damage to the cement by the etching acid.

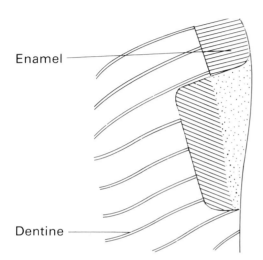

Enamel

Dentine

Fig. 9.29 Cross-section diagram through a sandwich restoration. ▨ glass ionomer cement; ▧ composite resin.

TUNNEL RESTORATION

The approximal cavity prepared on page 99 should be isolated with rubber dam if it has not already been done. A mylar matrix strip should be wedged in the interproximal space. It is usual to place a lining of calcium hydroxide cement on the axial wall. Some workers recommend the use of a conditioner prior to introduction of the cermet glass ionomes cement (p. 89).

A cermet should be mixed and syringed into the base of the cavity and the syringe slowly withdrawn as the cavity fills with cement. Excess material should be seen emerging through the approximal cavity. The occlusal access should be covered with a small piece of mylar strip and the cement allowed to set.

When the cement has set it should be carved on the approximal surface with sharp sickle sealers and on the occlusal surface with sharp excavators. The exposed cement surfaces should then be covered with bonding resin and cured with light for 15 seconds. A diagram of the completed restoration is shown in Fig. 9.30.

Some workers prefer to remove the occlusal 2 mm of cement and replace it by composite resin retained to etched enamel, using the sandwich technique. Whether this makes a stronger, more durable occlusal surface or just gives a better appearance is not clear.

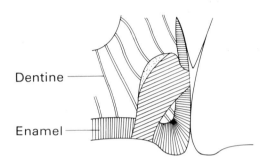

Fig. 9.30 Cross-section through a tunnel restoration.   lining;   glass ionomer cement.

Bibliography

Goldfogel M. H., Smith G. E. & Bomberg T. J. (1976) Amalgam polishing. *Operative Dentistry*, **1**, 146–150.

Hunt P. R. (1990) Microconservative restorations for approximal carious lesions. *Journal of the American Dental Association*, **120**, 37–40.

McLean J. W. (1988) Glass-ionomer cements. *British Dental Journal*, **164**, 293–300.

Robinson A. A., Rowe A. H. R. & Maberley M. L. (1988) A three-year study of the clinical performance of a posterior composite and a lathe cut amalgam alloy. *British Dental Journal*, **164**, 248–252.

Simonsen R. J. (1980) Preventive resin restorations: three-year results. *Journal of the American Dental Association*, **100**, 535–539.

Wilson A. D. & McLean J. W. (1988) *Glass-Ionomer Cement*. Quintessence, Chicago.

Wilson N. H. F., Wilson M. A., Wastell D. G. & Smith G. A. (1988) A clinical trial of a visible light cured posterior composite resin restorative material: five-year results. *Quintessence International*, **19**, 675–681.

10 Properties of rigid restorative materials

10.1 Introduction

In contrast to the plastic restorative materials which may be manipulated while they are in a soft state to fill cavities in teeth, there is a group of materials which must be shaped outside the mouth before the completed rigid restoration is placed into or onto the tooth. Where the restoration fits into a prepared cavity, it is referred to as an *intracoronal* restoration, whereas when it fits over a prepared tooth it is called an *extracoronal* restoration. The excellent mechanical properties of materials in this group lead to their widespread use for extracoronal restorations. The materials are less widely used for intracoronal restorations because it is easier, quicker and considerably less expensive to use a plastic restorative material.

Where there is a very large cavity in a tooth, it is preferable to fill the cavity with a plastic restorative material which has additional retention, e.g. from pins, and then construct an extracoronal restoration which protects the weakened cusps. The alternative of constructing an intracoronal rigid restoration, e.g. gold inlay, offers no protection to the weakened cusps and is considerably less retentive.

The rigid restoration is retained on the prepared tooth by the geometric form of the preparation, with the aid of a thin layer of luting cement which also prevents marginal leakage of bacteria or fluids.

There are two materials which have been widely used for rigid restorations for many years: cast gold alloy and a glass ceramic, dental porcelain. These two materials in modified forms may also be used in combination to achieve the aesthetic properties of dental porcelain with the strength of a metal alloy; the resultant metal–ceramic restoration is often referred to as a bonded porcelain crown. In recent years, polymeric materials have been used to make rigid restorations but their longevity has not yet been demonstrated. Another innovation has been the use of adhesive resins to bond rigid restorations to teeth. Until long-term evaluations are available, such procedures should be regarded as experimental.

With the rigid restorative materials an impression of the prepared tooth is taken in the mouth, so that a replica model can be made from the impression in a hard-setting plaster, dental die-stone, in the laboratory; the restoration is then constructed on the model. It should be possible to fit the restoration, which has been made in the laboratory, onto the patient's tooth with a minimum of adjustment; just how much will depend on the care taken in the execution of clinical and laboratory procedures.

10.2 Cast gold alloys

Cast gold was first introduced into dentistry at the turn of the century. The main attributes of this material are its strength in thin sections and its resistance to marginal breakdown and corrosion. It is particularly suitable for veneer restorations of posterior teeth as no more than 1 mm need be removed from the tooth surface. Because such restorations are usually made in the laboratory on models which give good access, it is possible to restore broken-down teeth to the natural contour with correct approximal and occlusal contacts. It would be very difficult to achieve this with plastic restorative materials intraorally.

The production of a cast restoration is an exacting and time-consuming technique. Because there is more room for error than with a simple restoration in a plastic material, it is necessary for the operator to pay particular attention to the adequacy of fit at the trial insertion stage.

These restorations rarely fail because of a fault in the material, rather because of errors created by the operator, or less often by lack of care from the patient.

Pure gold is not used for dental castings as it is too malleable, therefore it is alloyed. Table 10.1 lists some of the main types of gold alloy.

Type I is now rarely used, whilst type II is used routinely for intracoronal and single extracoronal restorations, particularly complete veneer crowns. Type III is occasionally used for onlays and partial veneer crowns, while type IV is more often used for them and particularly for cores of post crowns and for bridges.

A type II alloy contains about 75% gold, with silver and copper making up most of the balance apart from traces of platinum, palladium

Table 10.1 The main types of gold alloy for restorations.

Type	Description	Approximate gold content (%)
I	Soft	90
II	Medium	75
III	Hard	70
IV	Extra hard	65
–	Bonding (high gold)	84
–	Bonding (Au–Pd)	52

Table 10.2 Typical properties of type II gold alloy.

Proportional limit (MN/m²)	Tensile strength (MN/m²)	Hardness (BHN)	Melting range (°C)
160	345	70–100	920–980

and zinc. The exact amounts of each metal in the alloy and the colour of the alloy will vary with the manufacturer. Typical properties are listed in Table 10.2. This alloy is sufficiently malleable for it to be possible to adapt the thin margins of a restoration against the tooth to give a close fit; the procedure is referred to as burnishing. The alloy will retain a polished surface and will not corrode because of the high gold content. In recent years, alloys with a lower gold content and lower specific gravity have been developed to reduce the cost of such restorations. A typical alloy may contain 46% gold, with the balance being silver and palladium. Such alloys are more prone to oxidation during casting, and it is therefore very important not to overheat the metal at this stage. Dental technicians often find these alloys more difficult to work and polish in the laboratory.

A number of alloys have been produced to receive veneers of bonding porcelain. The most noble contain about 84% gold, with platinum and palladium forming most of the balance; these metals raise the melting temperature and lower the coefficient of thermal expansion of the alloy to match that of the ceramic veneer, a necessary requirement for successful bonding. About 1% of tin or indium is present to provide the essential oxide for bonding. After the dramatic rise in the cost of gold in the 1970s, alternative alloys which contain lesser amounts of gold or even none at all have been produced for bonding. The most successful have been the gold–palladium alloys. A typical alloy contains 2% gold, 79% palladium and 19% base metals, but no silver. Gold–palladium–silver alloys and palladium–silver alloys have also been used but discoloration of the ceramic may occur on repeated firing because of diffusion of silver from the metal to the ceramic.

With alloys totally from base metal, both nickel–chromium and cobalt–chromium, some problems have been experienced with unsatisfactory bonding and also with colour changes on repeated firing. It is essential that a compatible ceramic is used with the alloy chosen, and secondly that laboratory technique follows manufacturer's recommendations. These alloys have much greater stiffness than precious bonding alloys, making them well suited for long-span bridges, and their considerably lower cost makes them very attractive.

10.3 Dental porcelain

In the late 1960s, McLean developed aluminous porcelain which allowed stronger crowns to be made than were previously possible. The porcelain contains appreciable quantities of alumina, Al_2O_3, which strengthens the porcelain by hindering crack propagation. The major component of the porcelain is borosilicate glass with fluxes of potash, soda and borax.

A porcelain jacket crown is composed of three layers fused together. The innermost layer, which contains 40–50% added alumina crystals, creates a strong core but the alumina causes undesirable opacity; therefore, it is veneered with layers of dentine and enamel porcelains which contain considerably less alumina (about 10%).

A metal–ceramic crown is composed of four layers. The innermost layer is the metal coping, which is usually not less than 0.5 mm thick to achieve adequate strength. This is covered by a thin layer of opaque porcelain which masks the dark metallic colour but creates a bright reflective surface. It is veneered with dentine and enamel porcelains. Porcelains for metal–ceramic crowns have been specially selected by the manufacturer to have a coefficient of thermal expansion and melting range compatible with the appropriate bonding alloy. These porcelains flow more readily at high temperatures and may crystallize more on repeated firing than do aluminous porcelains.

Dental porcelain forms a durable restoration which does not corrode or dissolve. By suitable blending of porcelain powders during crown build-up a very good colour match can be achieved and the colour is stable. Glazed porcelain has a very smooth surface which does not encourage plaque to form on its surface. While porcelain has good compressive strength, it has low tensile strength; because of its brittleness it is liable to crack, particularly if there are flaws in the restoration. Porcelain jacket crowns, which are normally confined to anterior teeth, may fracture in clinical use but considerably less often since the advent of aluminous porcelain. Dental porcelain does not wear as fast as enamel and this may occasionally be a problem if the remaining natural teeth continue to wear, as may occur in a patient with erosion or a grinding habit. The crown will increasingly make a premature occlusal contact, particularly in protrusion; this may result in fracture of the crown. Dental porcelain is very hard but can be readily trimmed with a diamond wheel; trimmed porcelain cannot be polished although its surface may be made very smooth with abrasive rubber wheels. However, prior to fitting, the restoration is glazed, a process in which the surface layer is melted to form a smooth surface.

10.4 Cement lute

Rigid restorations are normally kept in place by a thin layer of cement lute which is usually about 80 μm thick. The set luting cement locks into the irregularities on the opposing surfaces of the tooth and casting. It also prevents marginal leakage and its thickness should be as thin as possible at the margins to resist dissolution.

The mixed luting cement must flow adequately when the restoration is being seated on the tooth so that the lute has a low film thickness. The cement should set quickly once the crown is seated, and achieve high strength rapidly. In addition the cement should possess low solubility, be non-irritant to the pulp and be light in colour to aid the appearance of porcelain restorations.

GLASS IONOMER CEMENT

As well as being used as a plastic restorative material, this cement has been developed for luting. The cement is presented as a powder and liquid. The powder is a glass virtually identical to that used for restorations, except that it has been more finely ground to give a thinner film thickness. A powder : liquid ratio lower than that for restorations is used to form a suitable creamy paste. The mixing may be done with a stainless steel spatula on a glass slab or waxed paper pad. Whilst the proportioning should correctly be done by weight, many clinicians add powder incrementally to the liquid until the consistency appears correct. Recently manufacturers have added the polyacrylic acid in vacuum-dried form to the glass powder; the resultant powder is mixed with water to initiate setting of the cement.

The mixed cement is applied first to the fitting surface of the restoration before being coated onto the previously isolated prepared tooth. The restoration is then fitted on the tooth and seated home; it is retained in position by the operator, or the patient clenching his teeth, until the cement has set. During this period contamination by moisture must be avoided. As the cement hardens, excess may be scraped off the tooth with a sharp excavator and interproximally it may be removed with dental floss; particular care must be taken to avoid gingival damage and bleeding. The margins of the restoration should be coated with two layers of varnish to prevent moisture contamination, because the cement is susceptible to solution in its early life.

The cement should be cleaned off the spatula and glass slab with a piece of wet gauze prior to setting, or afterwards by immersion in hot water.

The pulpal response to the cement is negligible. A great advantage of this cement is its adhesion to both dentine and enamel. It will also adhere to the oxidized surface of alloys used for metal–ceramic restorations and to the fitting surface of cast gold restorations that have been tin-plated, but few operators carry out electroplating as it is not necessary clinically.

The strengths of this cement compared with two other luting cements are shown in Table 10.3.

Table 10.3 Compressive and tensile strengths of luting cements.

Cement	Compressive strength (N/mm²)	Tensile strength (N/mm²)
Glass ionomer	150	9.3
Zinc phosphate	83	4.9
Zinc polycarboxylate	79	12.5

ZINC POLYCARBOXYLATE CEMENT

This cement is formed by the reaction of zinc oxide with polyacrylic acid and was developed in Britain a few years before the glass ionomer cement. It is used for luting and in its currently available presentation has better handling properties than when it was first marketed. The pulpal response to the cement is minimal and the cement adheres to enamel. The cement has no advantages over glass ionomer cement.

ZINC PHOSPHATE CEMENT

This cement has been widely used since the turn of the century. However, in recent years its possible irritancy to the pulp has caused some operators to switch to the more newly developed alternatives as their irritant effect on the pulp is known to be minimal.

The cement is formed by the reaction of zinc oxide with a 50% solution of phosphoric acid. Clinical experience has shown that when used carefully this cement provides a very effective lute. It is not adhesive to enamel or dentine; however, it can be difficult to remove the cement from tooth substance when a restoration is taken off as the cement interlocks into the irregularities of the tooth surface.

The cement is soluble particularly under plaque so a thick lute at the margin of a poorly fitting restoration is very susceptible to failure.

Cements based on the reaction of zinc oxide with eugenol have been specifically made for temporary luting. Their strength is lower than that of the permanent luting cements but adequate for the short time that a temporary restoration is normally in place. These cements are not suitable for permanent luting because of their low strength and high solubility.

10.5 Impression materials

Impression materials which are used to take impressions of prepared teeth must be very accurate and are usually of the setting type. They are based on polymers, principally silicones although polyethers and polysulphides may be used. The materials are frequently presented as two pastes which are mixed together in similar amounts. The operator then has a working time of several minutes to load the impression tray, coat the tooth and seat the tray correctly. After several more minutes the material should have set to an elastic, non-deformable state. The impression is then removed from the mouth and inspected for correct reproduction of detail and lack of voids. The impression should be dimensionally stable for some days, yielding an accurate model of the teeth. The most stable materials are the vinyl polysiloxanes (or addition silicones); however, the stability of the polysulphides, polyethers and condensation silicones decreases by a small amount after some days. Polysulphide impression materials have been widely used for many years and have proved to be very satisfactory. Conventional condensation-cured silicone impression materials have also been widely used, although the catalyst has limited shelf-life and the impressions can distort on prolonged storage. The most recent impression material is the vinyl polysiloxane; it has a very good shelf-life (over 2 years) and produces very accurate models even after several weeks' storage of the impression. Its superb dimensional stability makes it very suitable for taking impressions of multiple preparations. The cost of all these materials is high. Impression materials must be retained in a rigid tray with appropriate adhesive (silicone adhesive is incompatible with polysulphide material). Ideally an even layer of material in a custom-made special tray is recommended. However, in recent years there has been a trend to use putty consistency materials in standard trays with a wash of a low viscosity material over the tooth surface. In many instances, particularly for single tooth restorations in intact arches, this latter technique is satisfactory. Nevertheless, the special tray method is better for unusually shaped mouths or where a number of teeth are being restored.

Bibliography

Craig R. G. (1989) *Restorative Dental Materials*, 8th edn. Mosby, St. Louis.

McCabe J. F. (1985) *Anderson's Applied Dental Materials*, 6th edn. Blackwell Scientific Publications, Oxford.

McLean J. W. (1979) *The Science and Art of Dental Ceramics*, Vol. 1. Quintessence, Chicago.

Wilson A. D., Crisp S., Lewis B. G. & McLean J. W. (1977) Experimental luting agents based on the glass ionomer cements. *British Dental Journal*, **142**, 117–122.

11 Preparations for rigid restorations

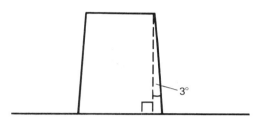

Fig. 11.1 The angle of taper of opposing walls of a preparation should be 6°.

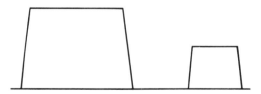

Fig. 11.2 Taller and broader preparations are more retentive when the angle of taper is constant.

11.1 Introduction

PRINCIPLES OF PREPARATION

Whilst it might be ideal to have a parallel-sided preparation for a rigid restoration, in practice it is impossible to achieve this as the preparation of the tooth is performed freehand. An undercut preparation must be avoided. Therefore, the operator aims to achieve a preparation with minimal taper. An angle of 6° between opposing walls has been considered ideal; in other words, each wall is at an angle of 3° to the long axis of the preparation (Fig. 11.1). In practice, this is unrealistic, and an angle between walls of 10° is regarded as acceptable. When the angle of taper was increased further in laboratory experiments, retention was substantially reduced. The length of the walls and the area of the walls are variables of the preparation which affect retention (Fig. 11.2). Another variable is the ability of the preparation to provide resistance to obliquely applied forces which tend to rock or twist the restoration; this resistance to displacement is achieved by placing axial grooves on the walls (Fig. 11.3). Retention is also dependent on the closeness of fit of the restoration.

PRELIMINARIES TO PREPARATION

A number of preliminary procedures and investigations must be carried out before the tooth is prepared for a rigid restoration.

It is necessary to ensure that dental caries and periodontal disease have both been controlled. Where there is evidence of previous disease, then the operator should be satisfied that diet and oral hygiene have both been modified as required and, further, that improvement has been maintained by the patient. The tooth should be examined clinically and radiographically to ensure that there is no untreated disease. In cases of severe periodontal disease, the prognosis of the tooth may be so adversely affected that provision of a crown is contra-indicated.

The vitality of the pulp of the tooth should be ascertained, and where the pulp needs to be treated this should be done before preparation for the restoration. Where the status of the pulp is doubtful, provision of a rigid restoration should be deferred until the status becomes clearer. A tooth with a history of pulpitis should be root treated before a crown is made.

Impressions should be taken for study models, to assess the occlusion, to allow a special impression tray to be made and to provide a guide during construction of the restoration.

11.2 Approximal inlay cavity

The clinical use of intracoronal cast gold restorations has declined markedly in recent years because the cost of producing such a restoration has risen out of all proportion to the limited superiority of the restoration over one using a plastic material.

The description of the preparation for an intracoronal restoration will therefore be confined to one which covers the main points. Other types may be derived from the principles employed and by reference to a more detailed text.

Let us assume that there is caries involving the distal surface of an upper second premolar and that a cavity for an inlay is to be prepared instead of one for a restoration in amalgam. The steps of preparation are:

1 Access to caries.
2 Determining size of carious lesion.
3 Keyway.
4 Approximal box. .
5 Removal of deep caries.
6 Bevels.

ACCESS TO CARIES

The first stage of preparation is to gain access to the carious dentine using a round or short-tapered tungsten carbide fissure bur in the turbine handpiece as has previously been described in Chapter 8 on page 100. The use of a tapered rather than a parallel-sided fissure bur avoids the production of an undercut preparation.

DETERMINING SIZE OF CARIOUS LESION

When access has been gained to the carious dentine, the cavity may be widened bucco-palatally until a sound amelo-dentinal junction is reached. This determines the bucco-palatal width of the box.

KEYWAY

It is usual to prepare a keyway, for not only does the fissure often need inclusion to take account of caries or a previous restoration but it also substantially contributes to retention of the inlay and its resistance to displacement. The keyway is prepared with a minimal taper of approxi-

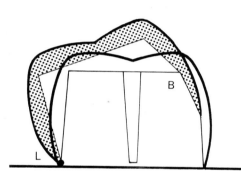

Fig. 11.3 Rotation of the restoration about the gingival edge lingually may occur if the buccal wall is short; this can be prevented by a groove on the approximal surface.

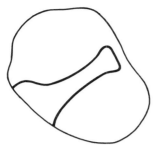

Fig. 11.4 The cavity is widened on the occlusal surface away from the box to form a dovetail in the natural contour of the fissures.

mately 10° using a tapered fissure bur, keeping the long axis of the bur in line with that of the tooth. The keyway is narrowest between the cusps and widens at the end away from the approximal caries to form a dovetail in the natural contour of the fissures (Fig. 11.4). As with the cavity prepared for amalgam, the keyway should be kept as narrow as possible and its depth should be only just into dentine except where the dentine is carious. Having prepared the keyway, the operator should dry the cavity to check that no caries remains in this part and that the cavity has slight taper in the correct axis. If the taper is incorrect it should be altered.

APPROXIMAL BOX

Attention may now be returned to the approximal carious lesion. In this part the cavity should be deepened with a round bur in the low-speed handpiece, in a similar way to a cavity prepared for amalgam (page 100), by removing the carious dentine at the amelo-dentinal junction. When all the carious dentine has been removed at the junction, the enamel wall may be broken out with a chisel and the margins tidied up with a gingival margin trimmer. A 10° taper is given to the preparation using a tapered fissure tungsten carbide bur in the turbine handpiece. Where a risk of damaging the adjacent tooth exists then it should be protected with a matrix band. It is most important to keep the long axis of the bur in the same line as that of the keyway so that the box and keyway have the same common taper. In inexperienced hands it is all too easy to create a tapered box and a tapered keyway which have different axes, preventing withdrawal of the wax pattern let alone insertion of the casting. The cavity should only extend as far gingivally as is necessary to reach an amelo-dentinal junction free from caries; similarly it is widened bucco-palatally only until the amelo-dentinal junction is free from caries. If any enamel is unsupported by sound dentine, then the enamel should be trimmed back with a fissure bur in the turbine handpiece.

A gingival margin trimmer is used to plane away unsupported enamel on the buccal, palatal and gingival walls. The stages of restoration of the tooth are made considerably easier if the buccal and palatal margins of the restoration are just visible from these aspects and if the enamel walls do not contact the adjacent tooth.

REMOVAL OF DEEP CARIES

Caries will probably still remain on the axial wall and it is best removed with a round bur (ISO size 012) in the low-speed handpiece. When the carious dentine has been removed, the cavity must be

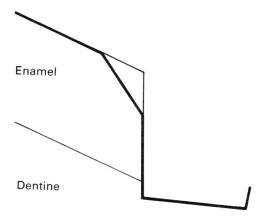

Fig. 11.5 The outer part of the enamel is bevelled on the occlusal surface to allow the casting to be finished to a thin edge.

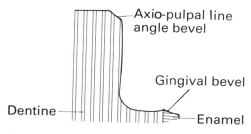

Fig. 11.6 Diagram of a mesio-distal cross-section through the cavity to show the bevelled axio-pulpal line angle and the gingival bevel.

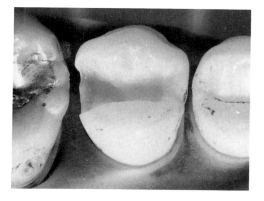

Fig. 11.7 The completed preparation which has minimal taper for an inlay in the upper premolar. Carious dentine has been removed from the axial wall of the box.

examined for undercut areas; undercuts at the amelo-dentinal junction should already have been eliminated. If undercut remains on the axial wall, it will be entirely in dentine and will be blocked out with lining cement at a later stage to give a tapered preparation.

BEVELS

The axio-pulpal line angle should be bevelled either with a tapered finishing bur in the low-speed handpiece or with a suitable finishing bur in the turbine handpiece. This increases the thickness of the subsequent wax pattern at a critical position.

It is desirable to prepare a bevel on the enamel margins, to allow the casting to be brought to a thin edge that can be swaged against the tooth should the fit be slightly imperfect.

In the narrow isthmus of the keyway on an upper premolar, the casting will normally naturally finish at an acute angle with enamel, so no bevel would be necessary in this part. However, to either side the cusp slope is much flatter and it is beneficial to place a bevel to approximately one-quarter to one-third of the depth of the enamel with a 12-bladed tapered finishing bur in the turbine handpiece (Fig. 11.5). The bevel should not extend deeper into the cavity as retention of the restoration is reduced. The operator may alternatively use a tapered fissure-cavity-preparation bur but great care must be taken to avoid overcutting. The outer margin of the bevel should be smooth and continuous to facilitate finishing of the restoration and to make a neat edge to the restoration. Where secondary fissures meet the bevelled margin, these deep grooves should be eliminated by saucerizing with the finishing bur. A bevel is not normally placed on the approximal walls because an undercut would be created, as most of the margin is cervical to the maximum bulbosity of the tooth. The gingival wall, however, can and should be bevelled, although it is difficult to do because vision and physical access are restricted (Fig. 11.6). The most suitable bur is a fine tapered Baker–Curson bur in the turbine handpiece. The gingival bevel is very important as it improves the fit of the casting where it is most critical. Since it is easy to damage the gingivae and adjacent tooth, other types of bur in the turbine handpiece should not be used to produce this bevel.

The preparation as described should have caused minimal destruction to the tooth whilst creating for the restoration a tapered cavity with sufficient retention and resistance to displacement without the need for additional grooves or pins. The completed preparation should appear similar to Fig. 11.7. Restoration of the cavity is covered on page 163.

11.3 MOD onlay preparation

The MOD onlay restoration is a particularly suitable restoration for a posterior tooth that is substantially weakened by large mesial and distal carious lesions. The cusps of such a tooth are susceptible to fracture if an intracoronal restoration is made. With an onlay restoration the cusps are reduced in height and then rebuilt in cast gold so that all occlusal forces are taken by the restoration. The load is then spread evenly over the entire tooth.

If the carious lesions are not very extensive, the tooth can be prepared to create a suitable shape for the cast onlay restoration, but where caries has destroyed substantially more dentine, the carious tooth structure may be replaced by a plastic restorative material, e.g. amalgam, prior to preparation for the onlay.

This restoration cannot be used where the buccal or lingual enamel wall of the tooth has been destroyed; and it is difficult, particularly for an inexperienced operator, to create a preparation with adequate retention on a tooth with a short clinical crown; in these cases the tooth is normally prepared for a complete veneer crown, which is a much more retentive restoration. Where there is adequate length of clinical crown, the onlay is a superior restoration to the complete or partial veneer crown, as it conserves more tooth substance and readily allows the vitality of the pulp to be tested. Further, the positions of the cusps are retained, which help in the construction of the restoration, and the margins are kept well away from the gingival tissues except on the approximal surfaces. The onlay is also appropriate for restoring root-filled posterior teeth with intact buccal and lingual walls, since such teeth are prone to fracture.

The procedure of preparing the tooth for an onlay requires particular care and skill; if the operator is careless, the restoration may be unretentive, and also an incorrect contour of the completed restoration may cause premature occlusal contacts.

The preparation of an upper premolar which has large mesial and distal carious lesions will be considered. In the first instance the tooth was prepared for an amalgam restoration, but after preparation the cusps were regarded as being unacceptably undermined such that fracture could well occur. The tooth was filled with amalgam; it provides an adequate short-term restoration, and it also makes a much better structural lining for a cast onlay restoration than cement, because it will not dissolve should the fit of the casting be imperfect. The preparation for an onlay is often performed on a tooth which contains a recently inserted large amalgam restoration, and it rarely involves the treatment of caries (Fig. 11.8); it is therefore very much a straight technical exercise and may be considered as a series of steps:

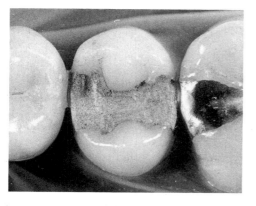

Fig. 11.8 A large MOD amalgam restoration in an upper premolar on which an onlay restoration is to be constructed.

1 Occlusal reduction.
2 Functional cusp bevel and shoulder.
3 Occlusal isthmus.
4 Proximal boxes.
5 Proximal flares and gingival bevel.
6 Occlusal bevels.
7 Finishing.

OCCLUSAL REDUCTION

The occlusal surface must be reduced so that the restoration is 1.0–1.5 mm thick and of the correct contour. Each cusp facet must normally be reduced by this amount and is conveniently done with a short cylindrical diamond or tungsten carbide bur (ISO size 010) in the turbine handpiece. To avoid unnecessary display of gold on the buccal side of the tooth, the occlusal surface at the margin is not reduced more than 1.0 mm. A series of grooves are placed on the occlusal surface (Fig. 11.9) to the appropriate depth; these grooves are most important for a controlled reduction of the occlusal surface. After they have been placed, the intervening tooth substance may be removed with the same bur. To avoid damaging the adjacent teeth, the approximal marginal ridges are left standing at this stage.

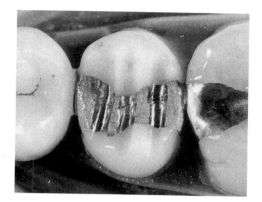

Fig. 11.9 A series of grooves have been placed in the occlusal surface as the first stage in the reduction of this surface.

FUNCTIONAL CUSP BEVEL AND SHOULDER

On an upper premolar in normal occlusion the palatal cusp is the functional cusp, and the onlay should extend onto the palatal surface to include the occlusal contacts with the lingual cusps of the lower teeth. These contacts should be located with articulating paper so that the preparation is not extended unduly far gingivally. The palatal aspect of the functional cusp is grooved to a depth of 1.5 mm, with these grooves extending just gingival to the occlusal contact. After the grooves have been placed, the intervening tooth substance may be removed with the same bur. At this stage, intercuspal occlusion should be checked visually and, if necessary, with the patient closing into this position on a strip of softened pink wax to ensure that there is 1.0–1.5 mm clearance; the thickness of the wax may be measured with calipers. Lateral and protrusive mandibular movements must also be examined. Any inadequate clearance should be corrected.

A shoulder 1 mm wide is prepared on the palatal margin of the functional cusp bevel. This shoulder provides more rigidity to the casting than does a chamfered margin and prevents distortion during the life of the restoration (Fig. 11.10).

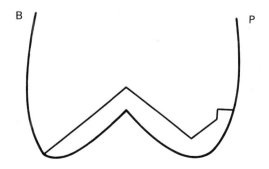

Fig. 11.10 Diagram of a longitudinal bucco-palatal cross-section (B–P) through the partly prepared tooth showing the palatal reduction of the functional cusp and the shoulder finish palatally.

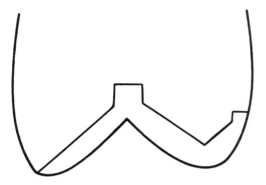

Fig. 11.11 Diagram of a longitudinal bucco-palatal cross-section showing the prepared occlusal isthmus.

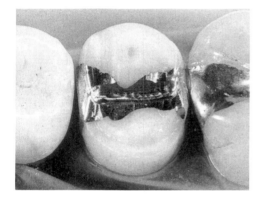

Fig. 11.12 The partly prepared tooth showing occlusal reduction, the functional cusp bevel and shoulder, and the occlusal isthmus; note that preparation has stopped short of the adjacent teeth to prevent their being damaged.

OCCLUSAL ISTHMUS

The isthmus is a channel which is formed to connect the mesial and distal boxes and is of considerable importance in giving rigidity to the casting (Fig. 11.11). The base of the isthmus should be placed at the amelo-dentinal junction; however, where there is a large amalgam core, the floor of the isthmus should be taken to a similar level even if it is actually still in amalgam. The width of the isthmus should not be wider than one-quarter to one-fifth of the distance between the cusp tips since further widening will significantly weaken the tooth or amalgam core. The isthmus should have a 6–10° taper between opposing walls and is formed with a short-tapered diamond or tungsten carbide bur in the turbine handpiece. As with reduction of the occlusal surface, the preparation is stopped short of the adjacent tooth (Fig. 11.12).

PROXIMAL BOXES

A small box should be prepared on each approximal surface with the buccal and lingual margins just within the existing amalgam restoration. To prevent damage to the adjacent tooth by the bur a matrix band should be placed around the adjacent tooth. Each box is prepared with a thinner short-tapered bur than that used for the isthmus. Each box should ideally possess a 6° taper and both should be aligned in the same axis as the occlusal isthmus; if they are not, one box will lock against the other. It is permissible to increase the taper slightly but it should not exceed 12°.

PROXIMAL FLARES AND GINGIVAL BEVEL

The outer parts of the buccal and palatal walls of the boxes are flared so that the margin of the restoration is extended to finish on enamel instead of on amalgam. Access for this is usually improved by removing the protective matrix band from the adjacent tooth. Where access is good, a fine sandpaper disc in the low-speed handpiece is suitable for placing the buccal and palatal flares. Alternatively a fine tapered finishing bur in the turbine may be used. The flares will eliminate any proximal undercut, but they should not be excessive, otherwise the width of the buccal and palatal walls of the boxes will be reduced and retention from them will be decreased significantly. The buccal margin of the flare should preferably not be extended more than 0.5 mm from the adjacent tooth, otherwise there is an unnecessary display of gold as well as unnecessary destruction of the tooth. Further extension would

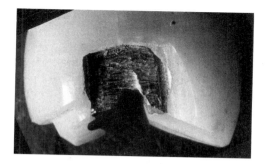

Fig. 11.13 The approximal box has been prepared, and a bevel placed on the gingival wall, merging into the proximal flares.

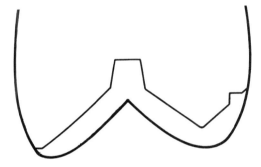

Fig. 11.14 Diagram of a longitudinal bucco-palatal cross-section showing the completed preparation with buccal and palatal bevels.

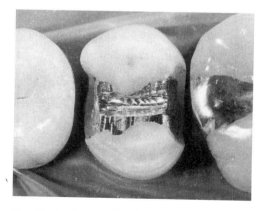

Fig. 11.15 The completed preparation for the MOD onlay.

only be carried out to reach enamel where there was a very wide amalgam restoration.

A tapered Baker–Curson finishing bur is used to form the gingival bevel, which should be continuous with the proximal flares (Fig. 11.13). The gingival margin of the preparation should be extended to finish on tooth substance instead of on amalgam, to eliminate any overhanging margin of amalgam and reduce corrosion between dissimilar metals. Where possible the margin should be supragingival to avoid gingival irritation.

OCCLUSAL BEVELS

The buccal occlusal margin should be lightly bevelled to protect the buccal cusp using a tapered finishing bur in the turbine handpiece held at approximately 90° to the long axis of the tooth; at each end the bevel should merge into the proximal flares. The palatal margin of the functional cusp shoulder is similarly bevelled (Fig. 11.14).

FINISHING

The preparation should be examined dry in a good light to check that each step has been carried out correctly and that the entire margin is smooth, continuous and defined; any errors should be rectified. The final preparation should possess a 6–10° taper; if there is undercut or excess taper, this should be altered. Further smoothing may be carried out with an abrasive rubber cup, wheel or point.

The internal surfaces of the preparation, which will be rough after preparation with a standard diamond bur, should be made smooth with a finishing bur in the turbine handpiece. Any of the following burs are suitable: finishing tungsten carbide, finishing diamond or Baker–Curson bur.

The completed preparation should appear similar to Fig. 11.15 and be ready for impression taking (page 171).

THE PREPARATION OF A LOWER MOLAR

With the lower teeth, the buccal cusps are normally the functional cusps, so the preparation is reversed compared with that on an upper premolar just described. The functional cusp bevel and shoulder is applied to the buccal cusps while the lingual cusps receive only a light bevel; a bevel is placed on the margin of the functional cusp shoulder on the buccal cusps and is made continuous with the proximal flares (Fig. 11.16).

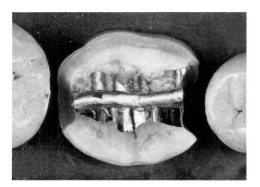

Fig. 11.16 A view of the preparation for an MOD onlay on a lower molar. The functional cusp bevel and shoulder is applied to the buccal cusps.

11.4 Partial veneer preparation

The partial veneer crown is indicated in preference to the MOD onlay where the palatal enamel wall of the tooth has been lost, probably as a result of the cusp breaking off. This crown is often referred to as a three-quarter crown. It may also be used as a bridge retainer. The preparation for the partial veneer crown can be regarded as a derivative of that for the MOD onlay, with the palatal surface of the tooth being included in the preparation.

It has become standard practice to build up the missing core of the tooth in amalgam, almost always with pin retention to prevent subsequent dislodgement of the core during preparation, or core and crown after construction. In a root-filled tooth, retention for the amalgam core is often gained by a post in a root canal (Chapter 15). If the operator has not placed the core, he should not proceed to crown preparation without examining the tooth for absence of caries and being satisfied that the core has sufficient retention. In recent years composite resin and glass ionomer cement have been proposed as core materials; there is limited evidence to show that they may be suitable but the casting must always extend beyond the margin of these restorative materials. Therefore, preparation is usually performed on a restored tooth and can be considered in the following steps:

1 Occlusal reduction.
2 Functional cusp bevel.
3 Axial reduction.
4 Proximal groove.
5 Occlusal offset and buccal bevel.
6 Finishing.

OCCLUSAL REDUCTON

This is similar to the preparation for the MOD onlay (page 153).

FUNCTION CUSP BEVEL

This too is identical to that for the MOD onlay. However, no shoulder is placed at the base on the functional cusp bevel (page 153).

AXIAL REDUCTION

A thin long-tapered diamond bur is placed in the turbine handpiece and three grooves are placed in the palatal surface of the tooth: one mid-palatal, one towards the distal and the other towards the mesial

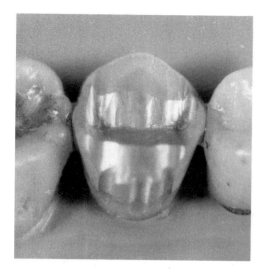

Fig. 11.17 Grooves have been placed in the palatal wall of an upper premolar as the first stage of axial reduction for a veneer crown.

(Fig. 11.17). At the level of the reduced occlusal surface the depth of each groove should be 1 mm, tapering to virtually nothing at the gingival margin. The gingival margin of the preparation must finish on tooth and not on amalgam to prevent corrosion of amalgam, to eliminate an overhanging margin and to increase retention. If it is possible to arrange for the margin to be supragingival and for the preparation to have sufficient length for retention then this is done. After the grooves have been placed, the intervening tooth substance is removed with the same bur. The value of the grooves is in achieving a controlled reduction of the palatal surface.

Next, the mesial axial reduction is carried out. A matrix band should be placed around the adjacent tooth to prevent accidental damage. The same long-tapered bur is used. However, if there is insufficient interocclusal clearance, a thin *short*-tapered bur should be used. The revolving bur is moved from the palatal towards the buccal and occlusal; a number of sweeps are required to achieve the desired preparation. It should not be done in one sweep as it is likely that insufficient coolant would reach the bur. The buccal margin should extend just beyond amalgam to finish on enamel; where possible the buccal margin should not be extended further than 0.5 mm from the contact with the adjacent tooth to avoid unnecessary display of gold.

After the mesial axial reduction, the matrix band is placed on the tooth behind while the distal axial reduction is carried out in a similar manner.

Because the axial reduction has been done in three stages, the corners where the separate facets join palatally are often ill-prepared and it is necessary to improve the axial reduction in these places.

The gingival margin of the restoration must now be defined and a chamfer finish is used (Fig. 11.18). This type of finish has become established for veneer preparations as superior to the bevelled shoulder, the plain shoulder or the knife-edge because: first, a definite margin is

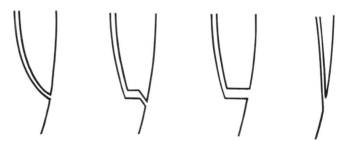

Fig. 11.18 The various forms of marginal finish for a veneer crown. *Left to right*: chamfer, bevelled shoulder, shoulder and knife-edge.

created on the preparation; secondly, it allows an adequate but not unnecessary bulk of casting essential for rigidity; thirdly, the edge of the casting is thin enough to allow adaptation to the tooth by swaging should it be necessary.

The most suitable way of creating the chamfer finish is to use a tapered finishing diamond bur with a rounded tip in the turbine handpiece. The bur has only limited cutting ability so it is relatively difficult to overcut with it. If a standard bur were to be used, overcutting would inevitably and readily occur, creating a spoilt preparation. As the chamfer is formed, the axial walls of the preparation are smoothed and the taper of opposing walls adjusted to give the desired 6–10° taper.

PROXIMAL GROOVES

To prevent palatal movement of the restoration it is necessary to place grooves, or even boxes, on the mesial and distal walls of the preparation. The groove gives the casting sufficient rigidity, is more conservative on the tooth and uses less gold than the box. The box is most often used when the partial veneer crown is being used as a retainer for a bridge.

The grooves are placed on the approximal walls with a thin tapered bur aligned in the long axis of the tooth; the bur should be centred about 2 mm from the buccal margin. It should not be closer, to prevent weakening of the buccal plate of enamel, nor further away otherwise the casting would be insufficiently rigid. Whilst such grooves can be placed with a bur in the turbine handpiece, the inexperienced operator will find it better to use a bur in the low-speed handpiece because tooth removal is less rapid. Some experienced operators prefer to use the low-speed handpiece with a speed-increasing head for the placement of grooves. The base of each groove should be just within the gingival margin of the chamfer and must not extend beyond. The groove should penetrate 1.0 mm into the axial wall at the occlusal surface of the preparation and it should be aligned in the long axis of the tooth. The palatal wall of the groove should be well defined to give effective resistance to palatal displacement (Fig. 11.19) and it should ideally be tapered at 6° to the palatal wall of the preparation (Fig. 11.20). However, the buccal wall is flared out to thicken, and hence strengthen, the buccal margin of the restoration; in doing this, resistance to displacement should not be affected. It does not matter whether the groove is placed in amalgam or tooth substance. The distal groove is prepared first; its axial alignment is checked after initial indentation of the surface of the wall, in case the groove needs

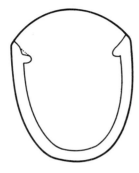

Fig. 11.19 The lingual wall of the proximal grooves should be well defined to give effective resistance to palatal displacement. The buccal wall is flared out to thicken the casting.

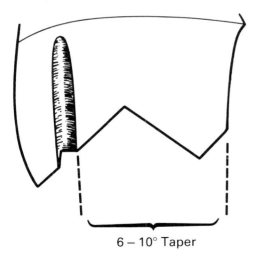

6 – 10° Taper

Fig. 11.20 The palatal wall of the approximal groove should be tapered at 6–10° to the palatal wall of the preparation.

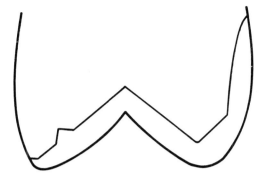

Fig. 11.21 Diagram of a longitudinal bucco-palatal cross-section showing the completed preparation, occlusal offset on the buccal cusp slope and shape of the completed restoration.

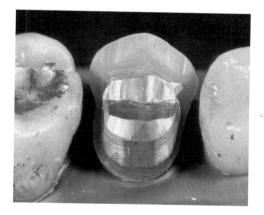

Fig. 11.22 The completed preparation for the partial veneer crown.

to be realigned. The mesial groove is cut second, as it is easier to align this to the distal than to do the reverse. After the grooves have been formed, they should be smoothed with a tapered finishing diamond bur or other finishing bur.

OCCLUSAL OFFSET AND BEVEL

To strengthen the restoration on the buccal side, the preparation is grooved on the occlusal surface of the buccal cusp (Fig. 11.21). This V-shaped channel extends across the occlusal surface to connect the two proximal grooves and is cut with the end of a short cylindrical bur held at 45° to the surface of the tooth; each wall of the channel should be about 1 mm wide. Then the buccal margin of the preparation is lightly bevelled with a finishing diamond bur to create a smooth, continuous and defined margin fron the mesio-buccal wall across the occlusal to the disto-buccal wall. The bur is held at approximately 90° to the long axis of the tooth. Excessive bevel is unnecessary and should be avoided because it causes an unsightly display of gold.

FINISHING

The preparation should be examined dry in a good light to check that each step has been carried out correctly. Any errors should be rectified. Rough surfaces of the preparation that remain should be smoothed with a finishing diamond bur and internal line angles should be lightly rounded with the same bur or a finishing tungsten carbide bur. Further smoothing may be carried out with an abrasive rubber cup, wheel or point.

The completed preparation should appear similar to Fig. 11.22.

PREPARATION OF A LOWER MOLAR

As with the MOD onlay, a functional cusp bevel and shoulder are created on the buccal cusps. Because of this the occlusal offset which is placed on upper teeth is unnecessary and is therefore omitted. A bevel is placed on the buccal shoulder and is made continuous with the proximal flares (Fig. 11.16); unlike the MOD onlay, an occlusal isthmus is not formed, as the restoration will obtain sufficient rigidity from the functional cusp shoulder and the lingual axial veneer.

11.5 Complete veneer preparation

The complete veneer crown in cast gold is extensively used to restore posterior teeth which have lost most of the natural crown through caries, fracture of cusps or wear. The restoration by encompassing the weakened remaining core protects the tooth from fracture. Since correct preparation of the tooth will only result in loss of enamel, the tooth is not further weakened. The complete veneer crown is widely used as a bridge retainer, and as an abutment for partial dentures because guide planes and rest seats can be incorporated. The preparation is relatively easy to carry out and the shape of the prepared tooth is highly retentive; this provides some leeway which can compensate for overtaper created by an inexperienced operator. The construction stage of the restoration is more difficult than for any of the restorations previously described, as there are no remaining enamel walls to guide the placement of cusps and surface contour. Because the entire clinical crown is usually covered by the restoration, subsequent testing of pulpal vitality is difficult, and recurrent caries is not readily detected until it is extensive.

The cast gold crown is now normally restricted to molar teeth where it is not readily visible, as many patients regard its appearance on a premolar as unacceptable and prefer instead the metal–ceramic crown (Chapter 13, page 188).

The preparation of a lower molar tooth will be considered. As with the partial veneer crown, it is standard practice to restore the tooth initially with an amalgam restoration to form a suitable core. The operator should ensure that the amalgam restoration has sufficient retention, usually achieved by pins, and secondly that existing restorations which are not being replaced in the tooth are unassociated with caries and are sufficiently retentive. If in doubt, it is better to replace than to find that there is caries or that the core falls out during preparation for the crown or during impression taking. In the author's view, large structural cores under crowns on vital teeth are best made from amalgam. There have been no long-term clinical trials into the use of composite resin as a core material, nor have there been clinical trials into the use of glass-ionomer or cermet as cores for crowns; the physical properties of these cements hardly suggest that they will be suitable for a complete core build-up. However, they may be suitable for limited parts of cores where dentine remains, and the margin of the casting must extend beyond the core material.

The preparation for the veneer crown may be considered in the following steps:

1 Occlusal reduction.
2 Functional cusp bevel.
3 Axial reduction.
4 Seating groove.
5 Finishing.

OCCLUSAL REDUCTION

This is similar to the preparation for the MOD onlay (page 153).

FUNCTIONAL CUSP BEVEL

This is similar to the preparation for the MOD onlay (page 153), except that no shoulder is placed on the functional cusp, and the functional cusp bevel on a lower molar is normally applied to the buccal cusps.

AXIAL REDUCTION

This is similar to the preparation for the partial veneer crown (page 156) but is additionally carried out on the buccal wall. In the case of a lower molar it is important that the taper of the lingual wall and gingival part of the buccal wall is not greater than 6° since the buccal wall is short because of the functional cusp bevel. It is necessary to check for the correct degree of taper from one corner to that diagonally opposite, since it is easy to leave undercut in these areas.

SEATING GROOVE

This is a single groove which is normally placed on the shortest wall of the preparation, the buccal wall on a lower molar (Fig. 11.23). The lingual wall of the groove should have minimal taper with the lingual wall of the tooth; the groove should be aligned with both approximal walls for the correct taper and to avoid undercut. It restricts the line of insertion of the casting, so allowing easier seating of the casting, and when the casting is in place the groove provides resistance to rotational displacement. The groove significantly increases retention and whilst this groove is not essential in every instance, it does make seating more positive. Where the preparation is short or retention is poor, several grooves may be used to increase retention considerably.

In the case of some lower molars with poor resistance to lateral forces (Fig. 11.3), the placing of grooves on the mesial and distal walls contributes significantly to resistance to displacement.

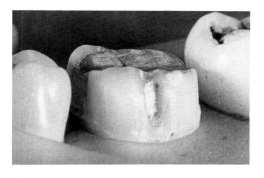

Fig. 11.23 The completed preparation for a complete veneer crown on a lower molar showing the seating groove in the centre of the buccal wall of the preparation.

FINISHING

This is similar to the partial veneer crown (page 159). The completed preparation is shown in Fig. 11.23.

11.6 Removal of cast gold restorations

Cast gold inlays may need to be replaced because of further caries in the tooth, cusp fracture or loss of the inlay from the tooth because of inadequate retention or resistance form. In the case of recurrent caries, carious tooth substance may be drilled directly if accessible. If it is not, the inlay must be cut into several pieces using a fine serrated tungsten carbide bur in the turbine handpiece. It is usual to divide the keyway from the box and then lever out the pieces carefully with a chisel or stout jaquette scaler. During division of the inlay, the operator should be particularly careful to avoid cutting enamel otherwise the cavity may be unnecessarily widened. In the case of cusp fracture it may be possible to lever out the inlay without dividing it.

When it is necessary to remove a gold crown, a cut should be made with a fine serrated tungsten carbide bur from the gingival edge to one side of the middle of the buccal surface straight up to and across the occlusal surface, taking particular care to avoid cutting the underlying tooth substance or core. A straight chisel (2 mm wide) should then be placed sideways in the groove and rotated; this will force the cut edges of the crown apart and break the cement lute. The crown may then be lifted off the tooth. With a partial veneer crown the cut would be made on the lingual side.

Bibliography

Shillingburg H. T., Hobo S. & Fisher D. W. (1974) *Preparations for Cast Gold Restorations.* Quintessence, Chicago.

Shillingburg H. T., Hobo S. & Whitsett L. D. (1981) *Fundamentals of Fixed Prosthodontics*, 2nd edn. Quintessence, Chicago.

Sturdevant C. M., Barton R. E., Sockwell C. L. & Strickland W. D. (1985) *The Art and Science of Operative Dentistry*, 2nd edn. Mosby, St. Louis.

12 Restoration with rigid restorative materials

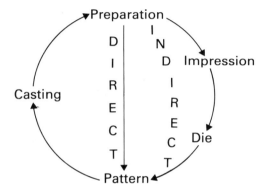

Fig. 12.1 Diagram of the stages in the direct and indirect techniques.

12.1 Introduction

Cast gold restorations are made by embedding a wax replica of the restoration in a refractory investment. On heating the investment mould, the wax melts and burns away before hot liquid gold alloy is forced into the mould, where it solidifies forming an accurate reproduction of the wax pattern.

For the simple restoration, the wax pattern may be formed directly in the patient's tooth. However, for the complex extracoronal restoration, the operator is able to make a better restoration by forming the wax pattern on a model in the laboratory; occlusal contacts can be seen more readily and additional wax can be added easily. Making the wax pattern in the tooth is known as the *direct technique*, whereas making it on a model is known as the *indirect technique* (Fig. 12.1).

The construction of an approximal inlay in the upper premolar will be considered first using the direct technique. This description will be followed by the construction of an MOD onlay using the indirect technique.

12.2 Approximal inlay

LINING

After preparing the cavity, it may be necessary to place a lining on the axial wall of the preparation, particularly in a deep cavity. This will also eliminate any undercut which might be present and reduce unnecessary bulk of the casting.

Suitable lining materials are a rapid-setting zinc oxide–eugenol cement, glass ionomer cement, zinc phosphate cement and zinc polycarboxylate cement. The cement is mixed to a stiff consistency on a glass slab and a small amount is picked up on the end of a probe and transferred to the cavity where it is placed on the axial wall. The material is tamped into place with a pear-shaped burnisher using a suitable separator (10% alcohol solution for zinc oxide–eugenol cement or methylated spirit for the other cements). Excess lining cement should be scraped away with an excavator before it has set and often no further finishing is necessary. However, if adjustment is required, the cement should be allowed to harden before it is trimmed with a tapered fissure steel bur in the low-speed handpiece without waterspray. Cements based on calcium hydroxide are unsuitable as they may be pulled away by the wax pattern.

WAX PATTERN

A proprietary matrix band and holder should be chosen; the Ivory No. 1 is often suitable. It is fitted round the tooth but no wedge is placed at the gingival margin. The isolated cavity is coated with a thin film of separating medium, e.g. 'microfilm' (Kerr, Romulus, Michigan, USA). The tip of a stick of clinical inlay wax should be heated slowly, well above a flame. As the wax softens it should be manipulated by the operator's fingers. Heating should be gentle enough not to cause melting of the wax on the surface, and is continued until the wax is completely soft. The tip of the wax stick is cut off from the remainder with a Le Cron carver, placed on the operator's finger and passed well above the flame before being taken to the mouth and forced into the cavity. Whilst the wax is kept under pressure with a finger, a wedge should be inserted between the band and the adjacent tooth at the level of the gingival margin of the cavity to compress the wax at the base of the cavity. The wax hardens as it cools rapidly. Excess wax may then be carved from the occlusal surface with a Ward's carver; the wedge is removed, the matrix holder loosened and the band rotated and slid out sideways so that the fit of the pattern in the box can be assessed. If the wax has incompletely filled the cavity the whole pattern should be removed and a new one made. If the pattern appears adequate, excess on the approximal surface should be carved away with a Ward's or Hollenbach carver. The wax pattern is then carefully lifted out of the cavity by engaging excess wax at the marginal ridge with a flat plastic instrument or a probe. The fitting surface should be examined carefully for sharpness of reproduction of the internal line angles and the gingival bevel. If reproduction is poor, the pattern must be redone; however, if reproduction is good, the pattern is replaced in

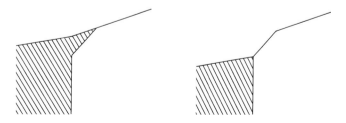

Fig. 12.2 The wax pattern must not be overcarved, otherwise there will be no fine margin on the casting. *Left*: correct. *Right*: overcarved.

the cavity and held there with a pear-shaped burnisher, while the remainder of the occlusal and approximal surfaces is carved with a Ward's or Hollenbach carver, or a small excavator. The pattern should not be overcarved otherwise there will be no fine edge on the casting to be adapted against the bevel (Fig. 12.2).

When the contour is considered to be correct, the patient should be asked to close his teeth together gently for the occlusion to be checked. Any prematurities indicated by a burnish mark on the wax surface should be adjusted; it is a matter of a few moments to adjust the wax pattern but of many minutes to adjust the subsequent casting.

The surface of the pattern should be made smooth by rubbing it with a pledget of cotton wool dipped in hot water and held in college tweezers. The approximal contact should be assessed as either adequate or in need of improvement by attempting to pass a piece of floss through it. A piece of wire at least 1 mm in diameter, with rounded ends and approximately 20–30 mm long, is gently heated at one end in the flame and then inserted into the marginal ridge so that it penetrates about 2 mm but not further, for risk of warping the pattern. In this example the wire should preferably be inserted into the ridge from the distal (Fig. 12.3), but if access is insufficient it can be placed vertically; this angulation is to allow the molten gold to flow readily

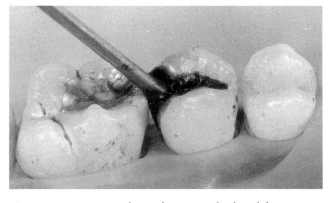

Fig. 12.3 A wire inserted into the marginal ridge of the wax pattern.

into all parts of the mould since the wire will form the sprue hole for the casting. After the wire has cooled, it is used to lift the pattern out of the cavity, so that the pattern can be examined for completeness and for fine margins both occlusally and gingivally (Fig. 12.4). A small amount of molten wax is then flowed onto the approximal contact area using a beaver tail burnisher to ensure that the contact will be tight after the casting has been polished; if the contact were inadequate,

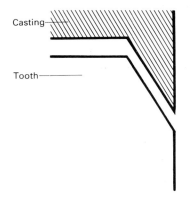

Casting

Tooth

Fig. 12.4 The gingival edge of the wax pattern must reproduce the gingival bevel of the preparation so that the casting will fit accurately.

a greater amount of wax should be added. The wire sprue-former is then placed in a piece of soft red wax or plasticine on a dappen pot to prevent the wax pattern from lying on the work surface and becoming damaged.

The wax pattern might have failed to come out of the tooth or broken during attempted removal, particularly if no separating medium had been used or the cavity lacked the correct taper, i.e. it was under-cut. The fault should be put right and another pattern made.

A temporary restoration is then made (Section 12.5, page 177) and the patient sent away before the operator takes the pattern to the laboratory for embedding in a refractory investment, which should be done as soon as conveniently possible after the patient has left to prevent distortion caused by a change in temperature.

LABORATORY PROCEDURES

The wire sprue-former and attached wax pattern are removed from the plasticine and inserted into an inlay cone; a ring of wax is formed around the sprue-former about 3 mm from the pattern by adding molten wax from a beaver tail burnisher (Fig. 12.5). This is to form a reservoir which prevents porosity in the casting. The casting ring is tried over the cone and the height of the pattern adjusted until it is approximately 5 mm from the top of the ring; the cone is then sealed to the sprue-former with wax. The wax pattern is coated with a special detergent to allow wetting of the pattern by the investment and to avoid entrapment of air bubbles on the surface. The ring is lined with absorbent refractory tape and then sealed to the cone with wax.

The refractory investment is mixed; usually a specific volume of liquid is added to a predetermined amount of investment powder. The correct powder : liquid ratio recommended by the manufacturer is im-portant for an accurate casting. Mixing is usually completed *in vacuo* to eliminate porosity. The investment is then flowed into the casting ring, which is vibrated to avoid air entrapment. When the ring is full, the investment is allowed to set undisturbed, preferably for more than 1 hour. The cone is removed and the sprue-forming wire is warmed over a flame so that it can be pulled out carefully with a pair of pliers. The mould is examined for loose or fragile pieces of investment which may be lying close to the sprue hole; any should be removed. The ring may then be placed in the furnace or left until convenient.

The temperature of the ring should be taken up to 700°C slowly in a furnace to allow the wax to melt, moisture to be driven off, the in-vestment to expand the correct amount and any residue of wax to burn out. This takes between 1 and 2 hours, depending on the equipment.

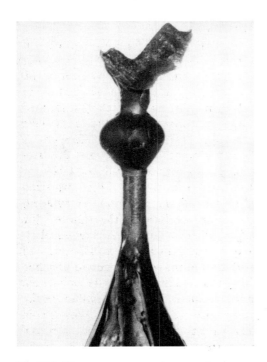

Fig. 12.5 The wax pattern on its sprue is inserted into a cone and the sprue is thickened to form a reservoir before it is covered with refractory investment.

Several grams of gold alloy are required for casting, which may be done in a variety of apparatus. The alloy is melted either in a flame or in an electric induction coil, and forced into the mould either by centrifugal force or by a combination of pressure and vacuum. When the molten metal has solidified, the investment ring is immersed in a bowl of water and the investment broken away from the casting, which is then examined for completeness of reproduction. The casting is next weighed and the investment is not discarded until it has been verified that no gold alloy has been lost.

The casting is placed in hot hydrochloric acid for a few minutes to clean off any oxide, after which it is washed. The sprue is cut off from the marginal ridge using a thin carborundum disc on a mandrel in the laboratory handpiece; the same disc is also used to remove the base of the sprue from the restoration. The marginal ridge is then smoothed with a medium sandpaper disc, and the contact area which may have been left rather rough by the addition of wax before investment is smoothed with the disc as well; any gingival excess beyond the bevelled margin should also be trimmed back carefully with the disc.

The occlusal surface should be worked over with a medium-sized round bur to remove any roughness but the margins must be avoided; a smaller round bur is used to define the base of the fissure. The approximal surface is then smoothed with an abrasive rubber wheel on a mandrel, whilst the fissure may be smoothed with a fine mounted rubber point. The approximal surface and marginal ridge are polished with a wheel brush using polishing soap, before the surface is brought to a high lustre using rouge on a leather mop. The fitting surface of the restoration should be examined carefully for any small spheres of gold caused by air bubbles in the investment. These should be removed with a sharp round bur to allow correct seating of the restoration in the tooth. Further adjustment to the fitting surface should be unnecessary. The restoration should now be ready for trial insertion and is taken from the laboratory to the dental surgery.

TRIAL INSERTION

The temporary restoration and any traces of its luting cement are carefully removed from the cavity, leaving only the lining in place. During removal of the temporary restoration and trial insertion of the permanent inlay, the operator should protect the back of the mouth with a sponge pack to prevent their inhalation or ingestion.

The inlay is taken to the cavity and inserted. If the approximal contact has been overbuilt, then it will prevent the restoration seating. The inlay should be removed from the mouth so that the approximal

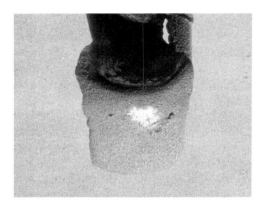

Fig. 12.6 The overbuilt approximal contact is seen as a shiny area of metal within the coloured aerosol marker.

surface can be coated with an aerosol marker (Occlude; 3M Health Care, Loughborough, Leicestershire). The inlay is reinserted in the tooth so that the adjacent approximal contact will scrape off the aerosol marker in the overbuilt area. When the inlay is removed from the tooth the affected area will be seen (Fig. 12.6) and it should be carefully adjusted by taking a small amount off the casting with an abrasive rubber wheel; this should improve the seating of the inlay. The contact is further adjusted until the casting seats, but it is important not to destroy the contact by overtrimming. Once seated, all the margins must be examined for fit and nowhere should there be a deficiency; if there is, the inlay must be remade. Any marginal excess which ought to have been removed from the wax pattern at the previous appointment can be trimmed away from the casting with a bur. The fine occlusal margins can be smoothed and worked down against the enamel with a pointed white stone in the low-speed handpiece. At the ends of the fissural grooves any excess may be eliminated with a small round bur. The occlusion should be checked; any prematurity should be located with Occlude, which marks polished gold more readily than does articulating paper, and then ground away with a carborundum point. Minimal adjustment should be necessary if the correct attention was given to the occlusion of the wax pattern.

If the approximal contact is insufficient and fails to provide resistance to the passage of a piece of dental floss, it is necessary to add to the contact area using gold solder. The inlay is removed and the contact area lightly abraded with a sandpaper disc to clean off any contaminant, such as grease. The contact area is coated with flux while it is ringed with graphite antiflux. A small piece of solder, produced for the particular alloy by the manufacturer, is placed on the flux and the inlay is held in a pair of soldering tweezers over a bunsen flame. It is heated until the solder melts and flows, when it is removed from the flame and allowed to cool. The inlay is cleaned in acid, washed and dried. The restoration is tried in the tooth and if it fails to seat home the contact is gently adjusted with an abrasive rubber wheel until it does. On the other hand, should the contact still be insufficient, more solder must be added. After polishing it should be impossible to observe the solder because the manufacturer matches the colour of the solder to the alloy.

The gingival margin of the restoration *in situ* should be examined with dental floss to detect any excess. If any still remains, the inlay should be removed from the tooth and the excess taken away with sandpaper discs and rubber wheels; this adjustment ought to have been done prior to the arrival of the patient. If the gingival margin stands slightly away from the tooth, it may be bent in by careful burnishing with a hand instrument after the inlay has been removed from the tooth. If the approximal surface has been adjusted it should be repolished.

An alternative method of assessing the presence of a gingival over-hang and the adequacy of gingival fit is to take a bitewing radiograph. Whilst an effective method, it receives criticism for exposing the patient to radiation.

The bevel at the base of the box is a valuable measure for over-coming deficiencies in technique. Should the casting be slightly under-size, the base of the box part will not fit against the gingival floor of the cavity; however, the knife edge of the casting will still overlap the bevel, thus reducing the size of the gap and exposing a smaller area of cement lute to dissolution by oral fluids.

To remove the inlay a scaler is placed under the approximal con-tact and pulled occlusally; this avoids damage to the margins of the inlay.

LUTING

The restoration is now ready for luting. The cavity is washed out, isolated and dried. The fitting surface of the inlay should be cleaned of polishing soap or debris and dried. The luting cement is dispensed onto the mixing slab and mixed according to the manufacturer's instruc-tions. The operator should use his cement of choice, although the author prefers glass ionomer cement. Further details have been covered in Chapter 10 (page 144).

The mixed cement is coated onto the fitting surface of the inlay, after which it may be coated over the cavity walls. The inlay is then inserted into the cavity and pushed into place with a pear-shaped burnisher positioned in the centre of the occlusal surface. The instru-ment may also be used to adapt the occlusal margins of the inlay against the enamel before the cement sets. A cotton wool roll may then be placed on the occlusal surface and the patient asked to bite hard together. This will force the inlay further into place and reduce the thickness of the cement lute. The patient should keep his teeth together until the cement has set.

Excess cement is then removed from accessible margins with an excavator while dental floss is used interproximally. The margins should be coated with two layers of copalite varnish to reduce dissolu-tion of the cement during the first few hours; this applies to all cements, although it is often only recommended for glass ionomer cements.

The occlusal surface should be polished with pumice paste on a brush, followed by whiting on a different brush and finally using

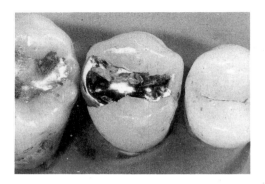

Fig. 12.7 The completed inlay in the tooth.

whiting on a rubber cup to give a superb lustre; this is similar to the procedure for polishing amalgam described in Chapter 9 (page 127). The margins should then be revarnished. The completed restoration is shown in Fig. 12.7).

12.3 MOD onlay

After preparation of the tooth for the onlay it is usually only necessary to insert a lining when an amalgam core is not present.

Because the entire occlusal surface must be rebuilt, it is much better and easier to construct the restoration on a model in the laboratory where access is unrestricted than to do it within the confines of the mouth.

SPECIAL TRAY

An accurate impression of the prepared tooth in the dental arch must be taken in order to form a model on which the restoration is made. This usually requires the use of a special impression tray, normally made from acrylic resin on a study model, prior to the appointment for tooth preparation. A special tray allows an even, thin layer of impression material over the teeth to minimize shrinkage distortion. It supports the material around abnormally positioned teeth much better than a stock tray and uses considerably less impression material. The tray should cover all the teeth in the dental arch to facilitate articulation of models. The periphery of the tray is extended approximately 2 mm beyond the gingival margins, but should be extended a further 2 mm in the regions affected by a deep overbite in some patients so that the models can be articulated. The tray is spaced over the teeth by 1–2 mm but should be close fitting at the periphery. The tray normally contacts three teeth around the arch (often the last molars and an incisor) so that it locates positively but cannot contact the prepared tooth. If adhesive on the surface of the tray was to contact the tooth, the resultant impression would be distorted and useless. The close-fitting margin of the tray is important to retain the impression material in contact with the teeth once the tray has been completely seated in the mouth. There must be no sharp edges on the tray as they might hurt the patient during insertion or removal of the tray. There should be a trial insertion of the tray to check that it is easy to place and remove without binding on the teeth or digging into the mucosa.

IMPRESSION TAKING

The impression is normally taken in an elastomeric material such as vinyl polysiloxane, because it is elastic and stable.

The adhesive compatible with the impression material should be coated on the internal surface and periphery of the tray as a thin layer and allowed to dry for at least 15 minutes prior to impression taking. It should not be allowed to pool.

The impression material is hydrophobic so the prepared tooth must be free from surface moisture. This is achieved by isolating the tooth, usually with cotton wool rolls, and placing a saliva ejector in the mouth; any bleeding from the gingival tissues is controlled first by placing a small pledget of cotton wool, then adding to this a small amount of alum solution. After several minutes the cotton wool pledget can be removed without bleeding. The gingival tissues should be packed away from the tooth with gingival retraction cord to allow a detailed impression of the gingival margin of the preparation to be recorded (Fig. 12.8). Several proprietary cords are available and a number of them contain adrenaline to reduce both gingival seepage and the volume of the marginal gingiva.

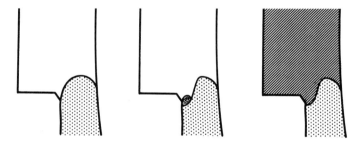

Fig. 12.8 The use of gingival retraction cord. *Left*: the gingival papilla is close against the gingival margin of the preparation. *Middle*: the cord is placed into the gingival sulcus to displace the papilla. *Right*: on removal of the cord, impression material is flowed into the space created by the cord.

Concern has been expressed about the use of gingival retraction cords containing 8% adrenaline; however, minimal systemic effect is caused when they are placed in healthy gingival sulci. Furthermore, rigid restorations should not be considered on patients whose gingival tissues are inflamed.

A thin cord should be placed into a dry gingival sulcus with the edge of a flat plastic instrument. It is only placed to the base of the gingival sulcus and must not be forced deeper in order to avoid damage to the epithelial attachment. The cord is left in place for several minutes, during which time it must remain dry. If any bleeding continues from the gingivae, the cord should be damped with alum solution. This must be subsequently dried before impression taking.

The elastomeric impression material of the operator's choice is dispensed onto the teflon mixing slab as recommended in the manufacturer's instructions, ensuring that catalyst and base pastes do not contact prior to mixing. The material should be *thoroughly* mixed with a broad-bladed spatula for the time recommended by the manufacturer. If incompletely mixed material is used, the resultant impression will be inaccurate and useless. After mixing, the material should be spread evenly over the slab to allow the escape of entrapped air. The impression syringe is partially filled with material before the remainder is placed in the tray. It is most convenient and economical to use a medium viscosity impression material suitable for both syringe and tray rather than to use a fluid material in the syringe and a more viscous one in the tray, particularly if a student operator does not have the assistance of a DSA; the use of a medium viscosity material is less likely to displace the retracted gingival tissue back against the prepared tooth than if a high viscosity material is used in the tray.

The retraction cord is carefully lifted out of the gingival sulcus by taking hold of a loose end with college tweezers, and immediately the tip of the syringe is placed into the gingival sulcus. The material is extruded slowly as the nozzle is moved around the tooth. The entire preparation is coated with material whilst care is taken to avoid trapping air, particularly in the corners of boxes. The loaded tray is taken to the mouth and rocked evenly into position, keeping cotton wool rolls from being trapped at the periphery; the tray should not be rotated into position as this may cause a deficiency of material. The tray is held in place until the material has set; the length of setting time is given in the manufacturer's instructions and may be verified by indentation testing for elasticity at the border of the impression. After the material has completely set, the tray should be removed carefully, usually by pulling down on one side of the tray, posteriorly, and then the other. The operator should avoid excessive distortion of the material as its shape might not recover completely. Pulling down on the handle alone is usually unsuccessful and also unpleasant for the patient.

The impression should be examined for general reproduction of the teeth with complete detail of all occlusal surfaces. Entrapped air is revealed as voids, which will subsequently fill with plaster and prevent the models from occluding properly; this error, unless of a very minor nature, requires the impression to be retaken. The impression of the prepared tooth should be examined in detail for complete reproduction, including the entire gingival margin and total absence of voids caused by air entrapment. If the impression of the preparation is imperfect it must be retaken since, by definition, an imperfect impression implies an unsatisfactory restoration. An unsatisfactory impression may be readily peeled out of the tray by immersing it in hot water.

A temporary restoration is now made; for details see Section 12.5. (page 177).

The operator must have an accurate model of the opposing arch and it should be unnecessary to take a further impression unless the contour of the opposing teeth has been modified since the impression was taken for the study model. It should be possible to locate the upper and lower study models accurately together in intercuspal occlusion, but if there is doubt the models should be marked in this position by referring to the points of contact on the patient's teeth. In some patients who have lost a number of teeth, location of the models is difficult and it may be necessary to record intercuspal occlusion in a suitable material, such as a proprietary occlusal registration material or fast-setting zinc oxide–eugenol impression paste reinforced with ribbon gauze.

Whenever an extracoronal restoration is being made, a facebow should be used to record the position of the upper teeth in relation to the hinge axis. Two layers of pink wax, which have been softened, are placed over the intraoral fork. This is then placed onto the occlusal surfaces of the upper teeth and may be steadied by the lower teeth. The facebow is adjusted to reproduce the hinge axis as accurately as possible. Whilst not all operators use a facebow, it helps in minimizing occlusal errors in mandibular movements and its use is essential when a number of restorations are being made.

After this, the patient may be sent away and the procedure is continued in the laboratory.

LABORATORY PROCEDURES

A layer of dental die-stone is placed in the impression to a level 2 mm apical to the gingival margin. As the stone begins to set, a tapered dowel pin is placed into the die-stone at the base of the prepared tooth with the pin's long axis in line with that of the preparation. Alignment may be guided by ball-point pen marks previously placed on the impression. Away from the prepared tooth the die-stone is roughened to aid retention of a subsequent layer of plaster. After setting, the die-stone around the pin is coated with a separating medium (dilute deter-

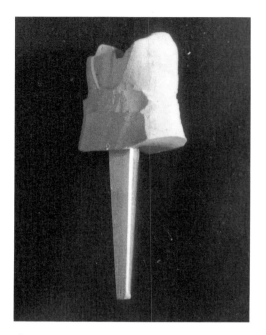

Fig. 12.9 The die must be trimmed to expose the gingival margins of the preparation.

gent), a small ball of soft red wax is placed over the end of the dowel pin, and dental stone is used to base up the model still in the impression. When this layer has set, the impression may be lifted off carefully and the model examined for imperfections, such as entrapped air. If the model is unsatisfactory it should be remade. A duplicate model of the prepared tooth is also made. The base of the full-arch model is trimmed until it is flat and the wax just exposed, before it is mounted on an articulator using the split-cast method; this method allows easy removal of the model from its mounting. The model should then be allowed to dry for some hours. The die-stone between the prepared and adjacent teeth is then cut through with a fine-bladed fret saw, taking extreme care to prevent damage to the preparation or the approximal surfaces of the adjacent teeth. The saw cuts should be angled to give a tapered die. When the saw reaches the base layer on the second cut, the model is turned over, the wax around the dowel pin is removed and by pushing on the exposed tip of the dowel pin the die should come out. The die-stone gingivae at the gingival margin of the preparation should be trimmed away with a scalpel to expose the full extent of the preparation; further away from the preparation, excess may be removed with a large bur in a handpiece; the trimmed die is shown in Fig. 12.9.

The surfaces of the preparation, apart from those within 1 mm of the margins on the die, should be covered with a layer of varnish to hold the model together, prevent abrasion and create space for the cement lute. The die is then soaked in separating fluid (Microfilm, Kerr, Romulus, Michigan, USA). Inlay wax intended for laboratory use (it has a lower melting range than clinical inlay wax) should be melted, preferably in a small heater rather than in a bunsen flame; the wax is then flowed onto the preparation with a small-bladed wax knife or Le Cron carver. It should be squeezed against the die to counteract cooling contraction and be built up in layers. When a coping has been formed, it should be removed carefully from the die to make sure that it has not stuck to the die-stone or varnish. It is then replaced and the die is put in the model to allow the occlusion to be built up using the wax additive method so that correct occlusal contacts in intercuspal occlusion are formed. The use of an adjustable articulator should allow correct contour of the restoration in lateral and protrusive movements of the mandible. The approximal surfaces should be contoured after the adjacent stone contacts have been trimmed lightly to allow for the minimal loss of gold during finishing and polishing. Finally, the margins are refined and the surface smoothed. A sprue-former is attached to one marginal ridge and the pattern is removed from the die. It should be examined for deficiencies; any present must be corrected.

The pattern is invested and cast as previously described (page 166). The casting is trimmed and polished on a duplicate die so that the working die is not damaged in the process. The restoration is then ready for trial insertion.

TRIAL INSERTION

This proceeds in a similar manner to that for the simple inlay (page 167). The approximal contacts must be checked and adjusted as necessary. The fit of the restoration must be assessed; deficiencies require remaking of the restoration, whereas excesses can be trimmed away. The occlusion must be examined for prematurities in intercuspal occlusion and in lateral and protrusive movements; any must be eliminated, although if the laboratory procedures have been carried out correctly, such adjustments should be minimal. The restoration should be repolished as necessary prior to luting, which has already been described (page 169). The completed restoration is shown in Fig. 12.10.

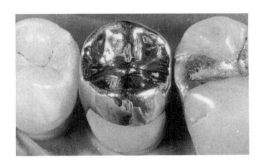

Fig. 12.10 The completed MOD onlay restoration on the tooth.

12.4 Special problems of dentures

These may be considered as: modifications of restorations which are being made prior to denture construction; and the construction of a restoration which must fit under an existing denture.

MODIFICATION PRIOR TO DENTURE CONSTRUCTION

In the partially dentate patient for whom a partial denture is indicated, the restoration of abutment teeth must be considered together with the design of the denture. The aspects of denture design which could affect the design of the restoration are guide planes, rest seats, reciprocal arms and clasps.

GUIDE PLANES

The contour of the axial walls of the restoration, particularly an extracoronal one, should allow suitable guide planes to be formed; this may require the alignment of the axis of taper of the preparation to be in a specific position, which would need to be decided after surveying the study model. The axial contours of the onlay or crown which abut the proposed denture would need to be formed by a carving instrument on a surveyor at the wax pattern stage.

REST SEATS

Where it has been decided to place rest seats, then sufficient tooth must be removed to allow room for the rest and an adequate thickness of casting to contain the rest seat. The rest seat should be prepared in the wax pattern because it saves time, effort and gold alloy compared with shaping it all in the casting; perforation of the wax pattern is a simple matter to rectify compared with that in the casting.

RECIPROCAL ARM

Where it has been decided to place a reciprocal arm within the contour of a crown, enough of the tooth must be removed to allow an adequate thickness of casting. The seat for the reciprocal arm is prepared in the wax pattern.

CLASP ARM

Where a clasp arm is to be placed, then the contour of the crown should allow the proximal part of the clasp to sit above the survey line, with the tip of the clasp able to engage a suitable degree of undercut for the type of clasp being used.

CONSTRUCTING A RESTORATION TO FIT UNDER AN EXISTING DENTURE

This most frequently involves the construction of an extracoronal restoration to fit under the rest and reciprocal arm of an existing metal denture. The tooth should be prepared in the normal way, with the operator ensuring that there is sufficient room between the prepared tooth and denture for the casting. An impression of the prepared tooth and dental arch, without the denture in position, is taken for a model to be used in the laboratory. After the impression has been taken satisfactorily and prior to fitting the temporary restoration, the tooth should be isolated and coated with a suitable separating medium, such as microfilm. Then a small amount of acrylic resin (Duralay; Reliance Manufacturing Co., Worth, Illinois, USA) (Fig. 12.11), which leaves no residue on burning, is mixed to a dough consistency and placed onto the part of the tooth which will be covered by the denture. The denture is seated home into the resin, which is allowed to harden. The denture is then removed and the acrylic resin wafer, which has an imprint of the tooth on one side and the denture on the other, can be lifted off the tooth. Excess acrylic resin at the margins is trimmed

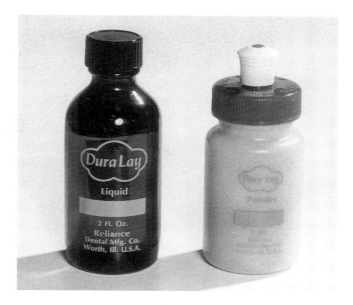

Fig. 12.11 Duralay acrylic resin for making patterns.

away so that it only restores the full contour of the tooth immediately under the denture rest and reciprocal arm. After being trimmed the acrylic pattern must still locate positively on the tooth. When this has been achieved, the acrylic resin wafer may be sent to the laboratory along with the impression. A model is made and the partial acrylic pattern is seated on the die. All margins and other contours of the restoration are developed on the die in inlay wax. The entire pattern must not be made in acrylic resin, first to avoid the distortion produced by its setting contraction (this particularly affects intracoronal patterns) and second to avoid damage to the investment mould as a result of thermal expansion when the resin is heated. This method produces an accurate restoration and does not require the patient to be parted from his denture.

12.5 Temporary restorations

While a cast restoration is being made, it is necessary to make a temporary restoration, which is used to:
1 prevent sensitivity of a prepared tooth;
2 prevent bacterial penetration of freshly cut dentinal tubules with consequent harm to the pulp;
3 restore occlusion of the teeth and prevent overeruption and drifting;

4 prevent damage to the remaining parts of the tooth, such as cusps which might fracture;

5 restore approximal contacts and so prevent food packing between the teeth because this would damage the periodontal tissues;

6 restore appearance.

The temporary restorative material should be easy to use, effective, non-irritant and inexpensive. Whilst a number of preformed restorations are available, the most versatile are custom-made using an alginate impression of the tooth prior to preparation as a mould. A material that has been widely used is Protemp (Espe GmbH, Seefeld, Oberbay, Germany), a bis-acryl resin. Another material, Trim (H. J. Bosworth Co., Skokie, Illinois, USA), a butyl methacrylate, is presented as a powder and liquid. Protemp has a base and two catalysts all in paste form (Fig. 12.12). Sufficient material to make the temporary restoration is dispensed onto a paper mixing pad; to this is added the recommended amounts of catalyst. It is thoroughly spatulated before it is inserted into the impression of the tooth with a flat plastic instrument, care being taken to avoid trapping air. The impression is reseated in the mouth and held in place until the material has become elastic and unmouldable. The impression is removed and the restoration inspected for entrapped air. Large voids will require construction of the temporary to be repeated, while small voids may be filled with a fresh mix of material after the temporary restoration has been removed from the tooth. The temporary restoration usually has a considerable amount of flash over the gingivae and adjacent teeth. This is carefully prized off with a flat plastic instrument and the restoration usually comes off the prepared tooth along with the flash. But care must be taken to avoid tearing the still delicate restoration. The restoration must be removed from the tooth while it is still elastic to prevent it becoming trapped. It is then allowed to set on the worktop; setting may be hastened

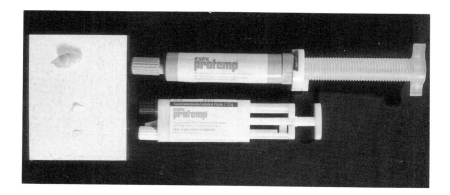

Fig. 12.12 Protemp temporary crown material.

without detriment by immersion in hot water. Excess material on the temporary crown at the gingival margins or under the approximal contacts of adjacent teeth is trimmed away after setting, most suitably with a medium grit sandpaper disc, and the restoration is tried on the tooth. Any gingival overhang must be removed to prevent irritation of the gingivae during the life of the restoration. The occlusion must be checked; prematurities in intercuspal occlusion and in lateral and protrusive mandibular movements should be located with articulating paper and eliminated; almost invariably there are occlusal prematurities to be removed. The temporary restoration should not be taken completely out of occlusion because over-eruption would occur.

Had part of the tooth been missing prior to preparation, this technique can still be used; an alginate impression is taken of the tooth before preparation, and after removal from the mouth the alginate in the affected area is removed with a large excavator before the temporary restoration is constructed. If the temporary restoration ends up slightly oversize as a result of overenthusiastic removal of alginate, it can readily be trimmed back to the correct shape with a sandpaper disc. An alternative method is to restore the defect on the study model with wax, soak the model in water, take an impression of it and make the temporary crown in the mouth as previously described.

After the restoration has been trimmed, the surface should be smoothed with a rubber wheel prior to luting with a zinc oxide–eugenol temporary luting cement, e.g. Temp-Bond (Kerr, Romulus, Michigan, USA). The cement is usually presented as two pastes, of which similar amounts are mixed together with a spatula on a disposable paper pad (Fig. 12.13). The cement is coated onto the fitting

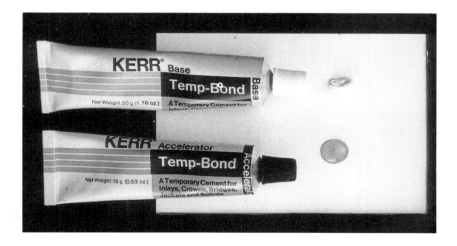

Fig. 12.13 Temp-Bond luting cement for temporary restorations.

surface of the restoration with a flat plastic instrument. The restoration is then seated on the tooth and the cement allowed to harden before excess is chipped away with an excavator. It is essential to remove excess cement interproximally with dental floss to prevent gingival irritation.

At the following visit, the temporary restoration is easily removed by placing a chisel at the gingival margin, pushing it against the tooth to drive its tip to the back of the chamfered preparation and rotating the handle; this is usually effective in breaking the cement lute, and the crown lifts off. Excess cement remaining on the tooth must be removed with an excavator and a pledget of cotton wool prior to trial fitting of the permanent restoration.

A temporary restoration is normally required to last a few weeks but many can last considerably longer. Where the temporary restoration is thin or exposed to considerable occlusal forces, it may break within a short time. Occlusal prematurities on the temporary restoration can cause loss of retention or its fracture.

Temporary metal crowns such as Iso-Form (3M Health Care, Loughborough, Leicestershire), made from a tin–silver alloy, are produced in a range of sizes for molar and premolar teeth (Fig. 12.14). They are not as versatile as custom-made plastic temporaries but are generally quick and easy to use; their margins can be trimmed, contoured and stretched. Occlusal prematurities can usually be bitten away by closing the teeth together before the crown is luted with temporary luting cement.

The use of preformed aluminium shells as temporary restorations which take no account of the occlusion has now ceased.

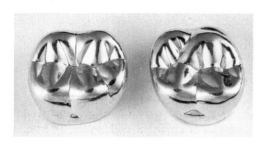

Fig. 12.14 Examples of Iso-Form temporary crowns. *Left*: for a lower molar. *Right*: for an upper molar.

Bibliography

Brown D. (1981) An update on elastomeric impression materials. *British Dental Journal*, **150**, 35–40.

Shillingburg H. T., Hobo S. & Whitsett L. D. (1981) *Fundamentals of Fixed Prosthodontics*, 2nd edn. Quintessence, Chicago.

Sturdevant C. M., Bartin R. E., Sockwell C. L. & Strickland W. D. (1985) *The Art and Science of Operative Dentistry*, 2nd edn. Mosby, St. Louis.

13 Ceramic restorations

13.1 Introduction

Dental ceramics are hard tooth-coloured materials which deteriorate little with time. The most widely used for anterior teeth has been the all-procelain crown, the porcelain jacket crown, which is retained on the prepared tooth by a cement lute. In the last 20 years, the metal–ceramic crown has been widely used for posterior teeth because of its greater resistance to fracture. More recently, labial veneers of porcelain retained to etched enamel by composite resin have been used for improving the appearance of discoloured teeth.

13.2 Porcelain jacket crown

An anterior tooth may be restored with a veneer crown of dental porcelain in situations where a considerable amount of the clinical crown has been destroyed by caries or trauma, or where the appearance is unsatisfactory. When a porcelain jacket crown is well made, it gives a durable and pleasing result; however, in addition to all the usual attention that must be given to the fit, contour and occlusion of a crown in metal, the appearance is dependent on the way the variously pigmented powders have been blended during construction. For this reason it presents a great challenge to the operator, and too often the results fall below expectations, especially in inexperienced hands.

The indications for porcelain jacket crowns have declined since the introduction of composite resin, the acid-etch technique and porcelain veneers. The porcelain jacket crown is the restoration of choice for restoring a very heavily filled and unsightly vital anterior tooth which has inadequate support for a labial veneer, because it gives a superior aesthetic result to the only satisfactory alternative, the metal–ceramic crown. Porcelain possesses good colour stability but its weakness is its brittleness. For the porcelain jacket crown this has been overcome to some extent by the use of alumina-based ceramics which were introduced in the late 1960s. However, fracture of jacket crowns is still a common cause of failure, particularly where there are errors in the shape and sharpness of the tooth preparation, as well as errors in the occlusal contacts of the restoration. The porcelain jacket crown is less suitable for young patients whose teeth still have large pulps, so these restorations are not commonly provided for teenagers. Fortunately, most fractured incisors in these patients can be adequately

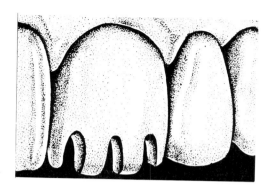

Fig. 13.1 Depth grooves are placed in the incisal edge to control the amount of tooth removed.

restored with composite resin retained by etched enamel. Usually the labial margin of the crown is placed in the gingival sulcus to give a good aesthetic result. However, in a young patient, normal gingival recession can cause the margin to become visible within a year or two; this is often unsightly and yet another reason for not making this type of restoration in young patients. Short clinical crowns provide inadequate retention of the restoration on the preparation, and thin teeth, particularly with a deepened overbite, may have insufficient room on the palatal surface for the necessary thickness of porcelain. Small upper teeth and most lower incisors rarely provide sufficient room for these crowns. Porcelain jacket crowns are not usually used on posterior teeth because they are too brittle. The restorations should also be avoided in patients who grind their teeth or have lost most of or all their posterior teeth. In these cases metal–ceramic crowns would be used because they have greater strength, although their colour match is likely to be less good.

Before treatment is commenced it is necessary to have established that the pulp of the tooth is alive and that there is no radiographic evidence of disease affecting the tooth. The operator should have study models from impressions taken at a previous appointment so that the occlusion can be assessed and also to provide a guide to the shape of the tooth during construction of the crown. Where it is intended to crown a number of damaged teeth or to reshape teeth extensively, a trial wax-up with beeswax should be carried out on a duplicate model. Reference can be made to this during construction of the crowns to ensure that they are of the correct proportions and their incisal edges are situated in the right place. A special impression tray should also be made.

13.3 Preparation

The preparation of a tooth for a porcelain jacket crown follows the same principles as those for a cast gold restoration. The mesial and distal walls of the preparation should have a 6° taper. The porcelain crown must be thicker than a gold crown for adequate strength, so the preparation is relatively more severe and the margin of the preparation is finished as a shoulder instead of a chamfer. The stages of preparation may be considered in the following steps:

1 Incisal reduction.
2 Labial reduction.
3 Approximal reduction.
4 Palatal reduction.
5 Finishing.

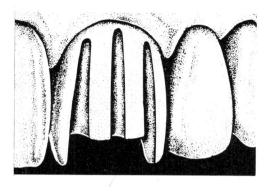

Fig. 13.2 Depth grooves are placed in the labial surface of the tooth to ensure sufficient tooth substance is removed.

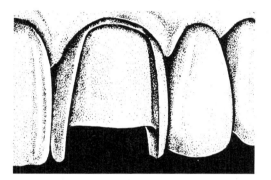

Fig. 13.3 The labial surface has been reduced but the gingival margin of the preparation has not yet been taken into the gingival sulcus.

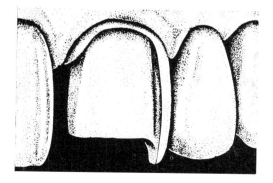

Fig. 13.4 The mesial approximal surface has been reduced and a shoulder finish formed gingivally.

INCISAL REDUCTION

Three grooves are made in the incisal edge with a long tapered diamond bur (555) in the turbine handpiece to a depth one-quarter the length of the labial surface of the tooth (Fig. 13.1). The intervening spikes of tooth substance are then reduced with the same bur, taking care to avoid the adjacent teeth. This shortening of the preparation enables the bur, which will be used to prepare the labial surface, to reach the gingival margin.

LABIAL REDUCTION

Three grooves are placed in the labial surface to the full depth of the bur such that the depth of each groove incisally is 1.3 mm, tapering to 0.8 mm at the gingival level (Fig. 13.2). These grooves ensure that sufficient tooth will be removed to give an adequate thickness of porcelain for strength and colour. If the original surface was convex inciso-gingivally, so should be the base of the grooves by altering the angle of the handpiece. If these grooves are not placed prior to reduction of the labial surface it becomes very difficult to assess how much tooth substance has been removed; and it is likely to cause a crown of incorrect colour to be made because the porcelain is too thin over an under-reduced core. The intervening tooth substance between the grooves is then removed to give a tapered reduction of the labial surface (Fig. 13.3); the width of the shoulder is 0.8 mm. The shoulder is then further extended until it is 0.5 mm into the gingival sulcus but it is not widened in the process. The operator will find it particularly helpful in preparing the shoulder to retract the free gingiva with a flat plastic instrument. As well as improving the visibility of the preparation of the shoulder, the gingiva is protected from damage by the bur.

APPROXIMAL REDUCTION

The approximal surface is reduced by burring away from the labial side and in doing so the bur is lifted incisally so that a number of strokes are necessary to achieve the preparation; this ensures that adequate coolant reaches the bur. Care must be taken to avoid the adjacent tooth and a matrix band placed around it provides some degree of protection. The width of the shoulder on the approximal surface should not be more than 0.8 mm (Fig. 13.4). The mesial and distal walls of the preparation should possess a 6° taper. With these walls as near parallel as possible, retention is significantly improved. The gingival margin of the preparation should be continuous and follow the gingival contour,

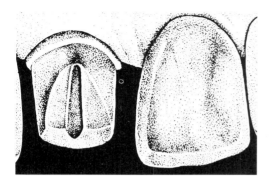

Fig. 13.5 Part of the palatal reduction has been carried out. A palatal shoulder has been created, merging into the approximal shoulders. A depth groove has been placed in the enamel of the small amount of remaining original palatal surface.

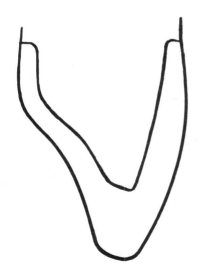

Fig. 13.6 A cross-sectional diagram to show the form of the preparation in relation to the shape of the completed crown which should reproduce the original shape of the tooth.

and this invariably means that the approximal shoulder rises incisally. The only exception is when there is an existing restoration with a subgingival margin. Indeed, the preparation should not be deepened to achieve a shoulder at the same level all the way around — though this may give a stronger crown; the gingival papilla will respond with chronic inflammation because of plaque accumulation.

PALATAL REDUCTION

A depth groove is placed in the midline of the palatal surface to a depth of 0.8–1.0 mm with the tip of the tapered diamond bur. The shoulder is then formed on the palatal side and merged into the approximal shoulders (Fig. 13.5). The palatal shoulder is usually placed supragingivally, unless the preparation is particularly short. The prepared tooth should be examined for slight taper; and any undercut, if present, should be eliminated, with particular attention being paid to avoiding undercut from corner to corner, e.g. mesio-labial to disto-palatal. The remaining part of the palatal surface is then reduced to the depth governed by the groove. Because this surface of the preparation should be concave it is better done with a small round diamond point in the turbine handpiece or a larger one in the low-speed handpiece. Clearance in intercuspal occlusion should be examined and it must be not less than 1.0 mm. This amount of clearance is also required in lateral and protrusive movements of the mandible and these movements must be checked even if there is more than adequate clearance in intercuspal occlusion.

FINISHING

The preparation should next be smoothed with a finishing diamond bur or other finishing bur, and sharp line angles rounded to reduce stress in the subsequent restoration. The incisal edge of the preparation should be bevelled towards the palatal side and in doing so the height of the preparation may be reduced slightly so that the final length of the preparation is two-thirds to three-quarters the original length of the labial surface (Fig. 13.6). Further reduction should be avoided as the crown is less well supported and the pulp is jeopardized.

The enamel margins should be planed with a 1 mm wide straight chisel or a binangled chisel where access dictates; this procedure removes spicules of enamel and creates a smooth margin to the shoulder on the preparation.

The finished preparation (Fig. 13.7) should be examined from several aspects for shortcomings, and any rectified. Frequently, inexperienced

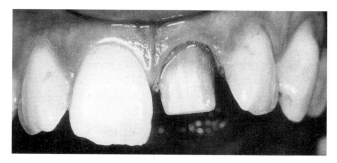

Fig. 13.7 The upper left central incisor has been prepared for a jacket crown.

operators become preoccupied about the need for a wide shoulder and overlook the undercut that they have introduced in creating the shoulder; there is no need to have a shoulder wider than 0.8 mm. Conversely, too much taper is undesirable.

Where the teeth are imbricated it is important to ensure that the preparation is not undercut by an adjacent tooth or it could be impossible to fit the completed restoration.

When the preparation has been completed, an elastic impression is taken, of which details have already been covered in Chapter 12 (page 171).

The shade of adjacent teeth must be recorded so that the restoration will be of similar appearance. It is advisable to assess the shade in good daylight but not in direct sunlight as it is too bright. Most operators use the Vita shade guide (Vita Zahnfabrik, Bad Säckingen, Germany) (Fig. 13.8) which has four basic colours: brown, yellow,

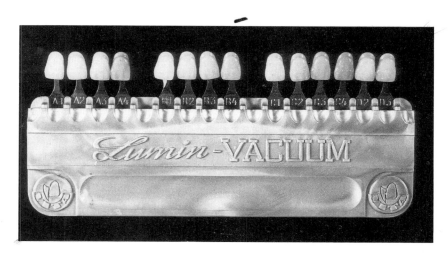

Fig. 13.8 The Vita porcelain shade guide has four basic shades lettered A to D; the higher numbers are darker.

grey and red, corresponding to A, B, C, D, with the lower numbers being light and the higher numbers dark. The operator should concentrate on the centre of the teeth, avoiding the cervical and incisal edge regions, to decide the basic colour of the tooth before determining the brightness. As general rules, teeth darken with age and the majority of teeth have a brown or yellow hue, so it is a good policy to assess the A and B shades for colour match before trying C and D shades. The enamel porcelains do not vary greatly between shades and it is normal practice to use the enamel powder which is suggested for the particular dentine. The tooth should be assessed for transparency of the incisal tip, whether it is as opaque as the shade guide or more transparent. Whilst the skilled ceramist and experienced operator may note subtleties of shade from cervical neck to incisal edge at this stage, the inexperienced operator/technician will find it hard enough to get the basic colour of the crown similar to that of the shade guide tooth, and specific characterization can be done after the crown has been tried in, using surface stains. When the crown is being made by an experienced technician it is very valuable if he can participate in taking the shade, or if he cannot see the patient he should be given full written details and a colour photograph.

A temporary crown should be constructed and luted into place with a temporary luting cement (page 177). Particular attention must be paid to avoid any gingival excess of crown material or luting cement, which might cause gingival irritation or recession.

13.4 Laboratory procedures

A model is cast in die-stone as has been described in Chapter 12; (page 173); the die of the tooth is removed carefully and excess stone trimmed to reveal the shoulder of the preparation. A sheet of platinum foil is swaged onto the die; particular care must be taken not to damage the model during this procedure. On the foil matrix a high alumina porcelain core is built up and fired. During firing the porcelain shrinks and may lift the foil from the shoulder, therefore the foil should be readapted to the model before further firing to ensure good marginal fit of the restoration. The build-up of the main enamel and dentine porcelain powders is critical to the colour of the final crown, and is particularly difficult to achieve without a great deal of experience (Fig. 13.9). After firing, the crown is ground with diamond wheels to adjust the contour.

When the crown is returned from the laboratory, with the platinum foil still in position apart from the gingival skirt which has been removed, the operator should assess the restoration prior to the arrival

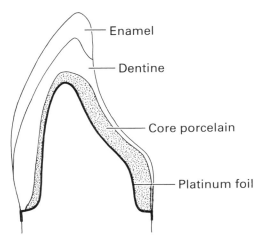

Fig. 13.9 Diagram of the different layers of a porcelain jacket crown.

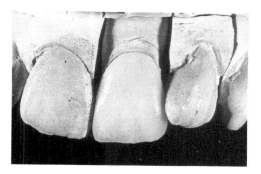

Fig. 13.10 The unglazed porcelain crown, still on its platinum foil matrix, on the model for checking prior to arrival of the patient.

of the patient (Fig. 13.10). The following should be examined: marginal fit and overextension, approximal contacts, shape, occlusion and colour. Any errors should be corrected before the patient arrives for trial insertion of the crown.

13.5 Trial insertion

The temporary crown is removed carefully from the prepared tooth and traces of luting cement must be cleared from the preparation before the crown is tried on the tooth. If all the laboratory stages have been carried out correctly, the crown should seat home fully; however, if the approximal contacts have been overbuilt, it will fail to seat. A trace must then be shaved off the affected contact with a diamond wheel in a straight handpiece with the crown held on the die for support; a diamond wheel is far more efficient than the previously used silent stone. The crown is retried and the procedure repeated until the crown seats home fully. The margins should be examined carefully with an excavator for full vertical extension, extending the full width of the shoulder but with the absence of overextension. Deficiencies in fit are difficult to correct, and unless they are of a very minor nature require the crown to be remade. Overextension, however, should be corrected by trimming back excess with a diamond wheel; for this procedure the crown should be held on the die. This trimming may need to be repeated several times before the overextension is completely eliminated.

The occlusion should be checked using articulating paper first in intercuspal occlusion and then in lateral and protrusive movements. Any prematurities should be eliminated using a diamond wheel with the crown seated on the die.

The incisal length should be assessed with the patient being examined in the sitting position. For this, reference to the original study model, or trial wax-up model, may be particularly valuable. Then the labial contour is assessed and adjusted as required. If the crown is undercontoured or an incisal angle is too rounded, the crown can be returned to the laboratory for the addition of more porcelain. Finally the colour is assessed. If the wrong shade has been chosen it is necessary to remake the crown. However, if the colour is very close when the tooth is examined wet, surface stains may be added to reduce the brightness by a light general application, and to alter the colour more significantly by heavier application, in particular areas such as the neck. Stains may also be used to simulate restorations, cracks and hypoplasia.

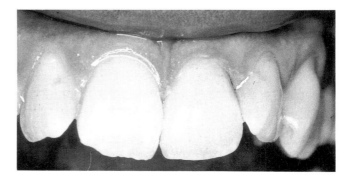

Fig. 13.11 The finished crown fitted on the upper left central incisor.

The crown is returned to the laboratory where it is stained as appropriate and glazed.

After glazing, the platinum foil is removed and any sharp margins smoothed with a rubber wheel. The crown is luted with a glass ionomer luting cement. The procedure is similar to that for a gold casting (page 169). The finished crown is shown in Fig. 13.11.

13.6 Metal–ceramic crown

This type of crown is considerably stronger than the porcelain jacket crown and it is therefore the restoration of choice for posterior teeth where a crown is indicated and the patient would not like a metal crown to show, or for anterior teeth where there is inadequate palatal clearance for a porcelain jacket crown; it is also frequently used as a bridge retainer.

Very often on a posterior tooth such as an upper premolar, the buccal cusp is restored in ceramic with the palatal cusp being in metal. The preparation of the tooth is a hybrid of that for a veneer crown and that for a jacket crown, with the palatal margin being finished as a chamfer while the buccal margin is finished as a shoulder. The transition from shoulder to chamfer occurs on the approximal surface toward the palatal side, so that no metal shows from the buccal aspect. The gingival margin should be continuous and not change levels or shape abruptly. The reduction of the buccal surface should be a little greater than that for a porcelain jacket crown. The long tapered diamond bur should groove the surface 0.2 mm deeper than the bur; at the occlusal of the buccal surface the depth of the preparation should be 1.5 mm, tapering to 1.0 mm at the gingival. This greater thickness compared with that for a porcelain jacket crown is to create sufficient room to accommodate a 0.5 mm thick metal veneer over which there

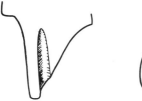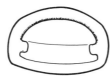

Fig. 13.12 Diagrams of a preparation for a metal–ceramic crown where extra retention is required from grooves on the approximal surfaces. *Left*: view from the approximal surface showing the groove at a 6° taper to the labial wall. *Right*: view from the incisal edge.

is enough ceramic to achieve a satisfactory colour match of the restoration. Some authorities have stated the need for a shoulder 1.5 mm wide rather than 1.0 mm wide, and while this increase may give an improved colour at the neck, it is unnecessary to remove so much dentine, and in teeth where the pulp is vital it may be potentially harmful. As these crowns are often placed on heavily restored teeth, the amalgam core must be well retained, usually by pins, since there will be little remaining buccal tooth substance to assist in retention.

On the occlusal surface at least 1.5 mm should be removed from the buccal cusp slope whereas only 1 mm need be removed from the palatal cusp, checking sufficient clearance in lateral excursions of the mandible as well as in intercuspal occlusion.

The resistance form of the restoration is improved by placing a seating groove, in the case of the upper premolar, on the palatal wall, which usually has sufficient dentine to accommodate it, whereas the other walls are closer to the pulp. However, if the tooth has a large amalgam core the groove may be placed on an approximal wall. Where a metal–ceramic crown is being made for an anterior tooth, the palatal clearance in intercuspal, lateral and protrusive occlusions should be at least 0.8 mm and the palatal margin is finished as a chamfer. If retention would be poor, particularly on a tooth which has suffered attrition in an older patient, it may be improved by placing grooves on each approximal wall in line with the labial wall (Fig. 13.12) provided that care is taken to avoid unnecessary encroachment on the pulp; this is usually not a hazard in teeth suffering from attrition or erosion. Such retentive grooves would not be placed in the tooth for a young patient lest the pulp be exposed.

On an upper premolar it is usual for the metal part of the crown to restore the full contour of the palatal cusp but only to provide a veneer approximately 0.5 mm thick over the reduced buccal cusp (Fig. 13.13). By the addition of approximately 1 mm of ceramic to the metal the contour of the buccal cusp should be correctly formed. The successful bonding of the ceramic to the metal requires a large surface area and the avoidance of sharp internal angles on the ceramic veneer. On the occlusal surface the ceramic should finish at a butt joint with the metal. The metal which abuts the ceramic should be thick so that it cannot flex and cause fracture of the ceramic. With all posterior teeth, it is important that cusps which have been built up in ceramic are supported underneath by metal to resist fracture of the ceramic veneer. With anterior teeth, the metal should be short of the incisal edge to allow translucency of the tip of the crown and the metal should be of sufficient thickness where it abuts the ceramic to resist flexion (Fig. 13.14).

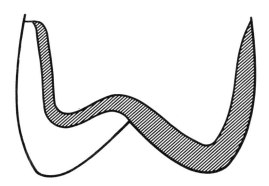

Fig. 13.13 Diagram of a longitudinal bucco-palatal cross-section of a metal–ceramic crown for an upper premolar. The palatal cusp is restored entirely in metal while the buccal cusp is restored with a 1 mm veneer of ceramic over a 0.5 mm layer of metal. The buccal margin has a shoulder finish while the palatal margin has a chamfer finish.

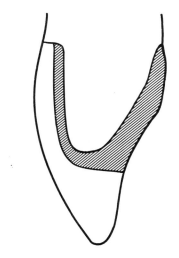

Fig. 13.14 Diagram of a longitudinal labio-palatal cross-section of a metal–ceramic crown for an upper incisor. The metal is kept short of the incisal edge to allow translucency of the tip. The labial margin is formed as a ceramic to tooth butt joint to give good appearance.

The labial gingival margin of the restoration looks unsightly if it is made of metal; however, it is possible to avoid metal showing by arranging for a ceramic-to-tooth butt joint. The casting is initially made the full width of the shoulder at the gingival margin but the metal is trimmed back 0.5 mm from the margin of the shoulder prior to the application of ceramic. A special ceramic which resists pyroplastic flow is used for the shoulder (Fig. 13.14).

After the crown has been made it is returned from the laboratory for trial insertion and the procedure is similar to that already described for a porcelain jacket crown. The exposed metal surfaces must be polished after glazing and before the crown is luted onto the tooth.

13.7 Removal of porcelain restorations

To remove a porcelain jacket crown, a groove should be placed in the middle of the labial surface using a diamond bur in the turbine handpiece with copious waterspray to prevent overheating. A straight chisel (2 mm wide) should be placed sideways in the groove and rotated (Fig. 13.15). This will crack the porcelain on the palatal side of the restoration and break the cement lute; the pieces of porcelain will normally lift off.

To remove a metal–ceramic restoration, a groove should be placed in the middle of the labial surface of the ceramic with a diamond bur until the metal sub-structure is reached. A fine cross-cut tungsten carbide bur should then be used to cut through the metal, taking care not to cut into the underlying dentine. A chisel is used to flex the metal and break the cement lute in a similar way to removal of an all-

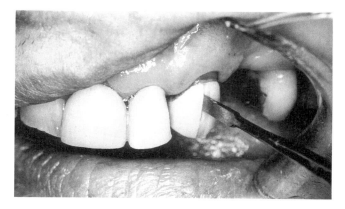

Fig. 13.15 A straight chisel inserted in a groove cut in a porcelain jacket crown prior to rotating the chisel.

metal crown; however, the ceramic veneer makes the restoration more rigid and the procedure therefore more difficult.

13.8 Porcelain veneer

For teeth which are discoloured by tetracycline staining or enamel hypoplasia but are otherwise structurally sound, the appearance may be improved by a porcelain veneer. This method involves minimal preparation of the labial surface of the tooth, followed by construction of a porcelain veneer, which is retained on etched enamel by a suitable composite resin. A porcelain veneer preparation is far less destructive to the tooth than a porcelain jacket crown preparation. It is therefore the restoration of choice where discoloured teeth need improvement of their colour.

It is essential that the margins of the veneer rest on enamel, so they are not suitable for patients whose teeth have suffered from erosion. During preparation of the tooth it is essential that the bur does not perforate through to dentine.

The preparation is best achieved with a round-ended tapered diamond bur in the turbine. A series of vertical grooves, no deeper than 0.5 mm, is made in the labial enamel, finishing as a chamfer at the gingival edge. The grooves are used to control the amount of enamel removed. The intervening enamel is then removed with the same bur. The edge of the preparation should form a clearly defined chamfer just short of the approximal contacts and approximately 0.5 mm into the gingival sulcus. The incisal edge should be given a 1 mm wide bevel so that the incisal edge is restored in porcelain. Failure to apply the bevel can lead to a veneer with a ragged edge. The entire preparation should be smoothed with a matching shaped finishing diamond bur or finishing tungsten carbide bur. The preparation should be dried to check that no imperfections exist. Errors should be corrected.

An impression of the prepared tooth is taken with an elastomeric material as has already been described for a crown (page 171).

Since the preparation has been confined to enamel, a temporary restoration may be omitted.

In the laboratory a model of the prepared tooth is made in a refractory material. The appropriate porcelain powder is built up on the model, which is then placed in a furnace to fuse the porcelain. After contouring and glazing, the refractory model is removed, the final traces being sandblasted off the porcelain.

When the veneer has been finished in the laboratory, it is returned to the surgery on a duplicate die-stone mode, for checking.

The patient's tooth should be isolated with cotton wool rolls to

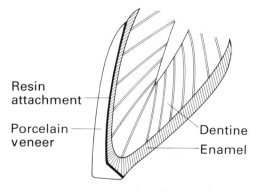

Resin attachment

Porcelain veneer

Dentine

Enamel

Fig. 13.16 Cross-section through a porcelain veneer on an upper incisor.

assess the fit, shape and colour. The fit and shape ought not to need alteration but can be adjusted by grinding with a diamond bur and polishing with a suitable abrasive rubber wheel. The colour may be slightly modified by varying that of the composite luting cement.

The tooth and adjacent ones should then be isolated with rubber dam retracted with a suitable clamp that does not impinge on the preparation. The tooth surface is etched for 1 minute with phosphoric acid, washed for 15 seconds with waterspray and dried for 15 seconds with compressed air from the 3-in-1 syringe.

The appropriate composite luting cement is selected, mixed and applied to the veneer, which is then seated on the tooth. It is cured by light for 15 seconds. Excess cement is then removed from the margins before the veneer is cured by light for a further 1 minute. The setting of these cements continues after removal of the light. The margins are finally checked for excess, which if present should be trimmed with a tungsten carbide bur in a low-speed handpiece.

The rubber dam clamp is carefully removed, and the rubber dam taken off. The protrusive occlusion is then checked.

When well done, these restorations provide a long-term solution to discoloured teeth.

Bibliography

Clyde J. S. & Gilmour A. (1988) Porcelain veneers: a preliminary review. *British Dental Journal*, **164**, 9–14.

McLean J. W. (1979) *The Science and Art of Dental Ceramics*, Vol. 1. Quintessence, Chicago.

14 Root canal treatment

14.1 Introduction

An important aspect of operative dentistry is the maintenance of healthy pulps in teeth. However, where a pulp is irreversibly damaged it must be removed and root canal treatment is carried out to retain the tooth, which would otherwise need to be extracted.

Root canal treatment embraces the removal of the pulp or its remnants from the tooth, the cleaning and shaping of the root canal space and the subsequent filling of the space. The purpose is to remove inflamed, necrotic or infected pulp tissue, which if it were to remain would cause inflammation in the periradicular tissues, usually at the apex. The long-term success of treatment is dependent on thorough canal preparation and complete obturation of the canal. Failures are usually associated with poor technique.

14.2 Indications

Root canal treatment is indicated when:
1 the pulp is irreversibly damaged;
2 the pulp is necrotic;
3 there is evidence of periapical disease;
4 previous treatment of the pulp has been unsatisfactory;
5 restoration of the tooth requires retention from the root canal;
6 the crown of the tooth is to be removed to allow the construction of an overdenture.

14.3 Assessment

It is important to examine the mouth carefully before commencing root canal treatment, so that there is no doubt about which tooth requires the treatment. If the mouth has been inadequately examined valuable information may be missed and the wrong tooth could be treated.

The jaws should be examined for a swelling which may be present in the region of the apex, and is usually situated buccally; with some long-standing infections there may be a swelling remote from the tooth. The swelling and the offending tooth are likely to be tender and this indicates acute periapical disease, i.e. an abscess. The jaws should also be examined for a sinus tract indicative of a chronic discharging infection and where present its direction should be investigated by inserting a gutta-percha point and taking a radiograph to verify which tooth is the cause.

The periodontal condition of the tooth requiring treatment should be assessed and treated as necessary. Only advanced periodontal disease is a contra-indication to root canal treatment. If there is a carious lesion in the tooth requiring treatment, it must be treated first to prevent bacterial contamination of the root canal during root canal treatment. The tooth should be examined carefully for fractures and any which are found investigated before commencing root treatment. The vitality of the pulp must be assessed with an electric pulp tester and thermal tests before treatment is undertaken.

An intraoral periapical radiograph of the tooth must be taken for preoperative assessment, preferably by the paralleling technique because this view reduces distortion, is reproducible and the approximate length of the tooth can be measured. The radiograph should be examined for:

1 number of roots and curvature;
2 presence and size of canals;
3 position and size of pulp chamber;
4 evidence of periradicular disease, which usually affects the periapical tissues but may affect the side of the root if a large lateral canal is present;
5 resorption of the root;
6 evidence of previous treatment;
7 stage of root development in a young person.

14.4 Equipment

Specially designed root canal instruments are used to shape the root canal. The basic design of a K-file is shown in Fig. 14.1. It has a pointed tip which is not intended for cutting, a working part with sharp cutting flutes, a smooth shaft and a handle. The taper of the working part is constant at 0.02 mm per millimetre over its length of approximately 16 mm. The size of the instrument is taken from the diameter of the working part adjacent to the tip, and is usually quoted

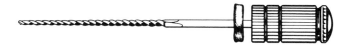

Fig. 14.1 Diagram of a standardized instrument. The taper of the working part is 0.02 mm per millimetre over its approximate length of 16 mm.

Table 14.1 Sizes of files available, diameter of instruments at tip and ISO colours

Size	Tip diameter (mm)	ISO colour
06	0.06	Pink
08	0.08	Grey
10	0.10	Purple
15	0.15	White
20	0.20	Yellow
25	0.25	Red
30	0.30	Blue
35	0.35	Green
40	0.40	Black
45	0.45	White
50	0.50	Yellow
55	0.55	Red
60	0.60	Blue
70	0.70	Green
80	0.80	Black
90	0.90	White
100	1.00	Yellow
110	1.10	Red
120	1.20	Blue
130	1.30	Green
140	1.40	Black

in hundredths of a millimetre. Sizes available are given in Table 14.1. The size of an instrument is stamped on the handle, which is usually colour coded. Unfortunately not all manufacturers have adopted the ISO colour coding, but provided that the instruments of only one manufacturer are used it is not confusing for the operator. Six basic colours are used in sequence and recur in the larger sizes but the difference in size is readily seen. Instruments are available in different lengths, to cater for molars with restricted access and, at the other extreme, canines with long roots. The length of the instrument from tip to base of the handle is variable in the range 20–30 mm, the exact length depending on the manufacturer; however, the usual length is 25 mm.

A marker stop is used on the shaft of the instrument to control its depth of insertion into the tooth; the marker is usually a disc of silicone rubber which the operator can adjust.

The K-file will cut dentine in a push or pull action, hence the name 'file'. It will also cut dentine with a turning action so it has wide application for preparing canals.

Alternative instruments for preparing canals are reamers, K-flex

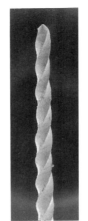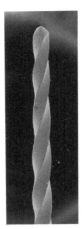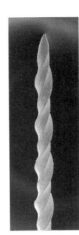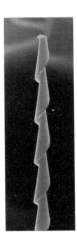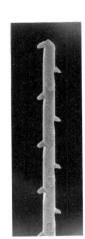

Fig. 14.2 Instruments for preparing root canals and removing pulps. *Left to right*: K-file, reamer, K-flex file, Hedstrom file, and barbed broach for pulp removal.

files (Kerr, Romulus, Michigan, USA), and Hedstrom files (Fig. 14.2). Reamers are similar to K-files but have fewer cutting flutes per unit length and are intended for cutting with a turning action. They are not now so widely used because of the greater use of a filing action which is indicated for curved canals. K-flex files are relatively newer instruments with increased flexibility and very sharp cutting flutes; they are used in a similar way to K-files. Hedstrom files only cut in a pull motion but they remove dentine very rapidly; these files must not be screwed into a canal, for such abuse invites fracture of the thin shaft should it bind. All these cutting instruments are made from stainless steel.

The pulp in a wide root canal can be removed with a barbed broach (Fig. 14.2) but this type of instrument should not be used in a fine canal in case it binds; barbed broaches are therefore not widely used in

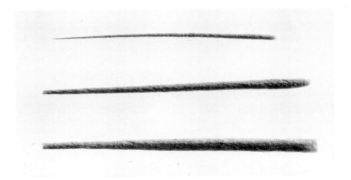

Fig. 14.3 Three sizes of paper points for drying root canals.

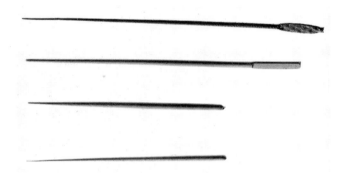

Fig. 14.4 Gutta-percha cones for filling root canals. *Top to bottom*: size 25 standardized, size 40 standardized, wide accessory point and fine accessory point.

the treatment of mature teeth in adults. Root canals can be dried with paper points (Fig. 14.3) which are supplied sterile in various sizes.

Most root canals are normally filled with gutta-percha cones. These are produced in a range of sizes that nominally correspond to instrument sizes (Fig. 14.4). Also, finer, stiffer and more tapered accessory

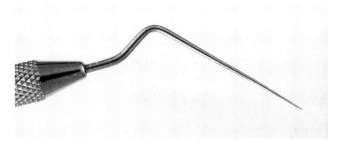

Fig. 14.5 A fine lateral spreader.

points are available for secondary filling of the canal by lateral condensation. To condense the root filling, a lateral spreader is used; it is a fine pointed springy piece of stainless steel either on a long handle for ease of use (Fig. 14.5) or with a short handle, a finger spreader, for use in fine canals in molars. It must not be bent or heated in a flame, otherwise it is more likely to remove the filling than condense it.

14.5 Stages of treatment

These may be considered as follows:
1 Isolation.
2 Access.

3 Canal length.
4 Preparation.
5 Irrigation.
6 Medication.
7 Temporary restoration.
8 Filling.

Whatever the condition of the pulp or periapical tissues, the stages of treatment are essentially the same. Where the radicular pulp is *vital*, treatment in one visit is possible and becoming increasingly practised. Where there is periapical disease, treatment is normally spread over two visits with canal preparation being completed at the first visit; should there be a flare-up of a chronic periapical lesion after canal preparation, the root canal can be used for drainage.

ISOLATION

A saliva-free working environment is important for all operative dentistry, but adequate isolation of the tooth being treated is even more necessary for root canal treatment, first to prevent or stop further infection of the pulp, secondly to keep irrigating solutions out of the mouth, and thirdly to prevent root canal instruments from being inhaled or ingested. This medico-legal reason for adequate isolation is most important and has almost overshadowed the others. Should a patient inhale or ingest an instrument, the operator will have no defence against an allegation of negligence if he had not taken any precautions. For the majority of root canal treatments, rubber dam can be retained solely on the tooth being treated and this simplifies its application. The tooth should be isolated before the access cavity is prepared. Rubber dam application is considered in Chapter 16 (page 253). The use of less satisfactory forms of isolation, such as cotton wool rolls or sponges, is not an adequate alternative in the view of the author. Root treatment should be carried out using an aseptic technique. The tooth surface should be disinfected after isolation with a pledget of cotton wool soaked in disinfectant, e.g. sodium hypochlorite solution. The root canal instruments should be presterilized in an autoclave and kept in a suitable stand (Fig. 14.6).

ACCESS

The entire roof of the pulp chamber must be removed to allow complete cleaning of the pulp chamber and to allow root canal files to pass along the canals without being bent excessively. The position and shape of the cavity depend on the particular tooth being treated (Figs

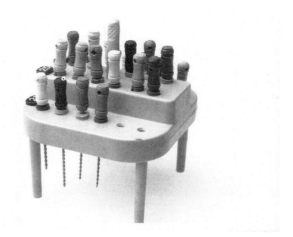

Fig. 14.6 Root canal files in an autoclavable stand.

14.7 & 14.8). However, it is rare that a cavity prepared during the treatment of caries is in the correct position. Whilst it may be tempting to use such a cavity to conserve tooth substance, the pulp chamber cannot be cleaned properly, root canal files are very likely to break because of excessive bending and the apical part of the root canal will be prepared inadequately and incorrectly, making subsequent correction very difficult. Poor access to the pulp chamber may prevent all the canals from being found; in a lower incisor a second canal can be missed if the access cavity is inadequate (Fig. 14.9).

The preoperative radiograph should be assessed carefully for the size and position of the pulp chamber. It may be large, making its discovery easy, or it may be small and quite far apically as a result of the deposition of reactionary dentine. By placing the bur on the preoperative radiograph taken by the paralleling technique, its distance into the tooth to reach the pulp chamber can be assessed as well as its angulation in a mesio-distal plane.

For an upper incisor the access cavity is prepared on the palatal surface and is triangular in outline with its base close to the incisal edge (Fig. 14.7). The enamel should be drilled away with a bur in the turbine handpiece. The dentine should then be removed with a round bur (ISO size 012) in the low-speed handpiece because the bur is longer and the operator has greater feel. On reaching the pulp chamber the bur will fall into the pulp; the roof is then removed by *pull* strokes with the bur. Push strokes must be avoided to prevent gouging of the labial wall of the pulp chamber (Fig. 14.9); excessive gouging can lead to perforation of the labial wall. The completed access cavity should

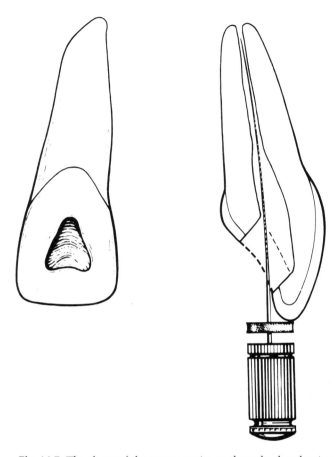

Fig. 14.7 The shape of the access cavity to the pulp chamber in an upper incisor.

be funnel-shaped and by solely using round burs no ledges should be formed in the walls of the pulp chamber. Where the pulp chamber is small and difficult to find, the operator must not drill blindly but refer to the radiograph. The angulation of the bur in the long axis should be verified by checking that there is no deviation mesially or distally. The labio-palatal position is guided by the jaws of the rubber dam clamp. If the head of the handpiece hits the incisal edge, either a normal length bur in a miniature head should be used or an extra-long bur in the standard head. The access cavity on posterior teeth is made through a specific part of the occlusal surface. Reference should be made to a textbook of endodontics.

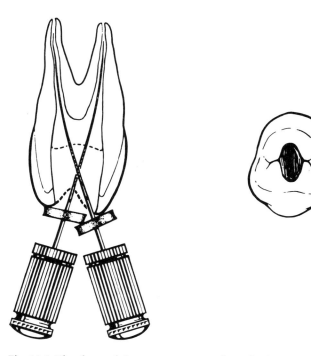

Fig. 14.8 The shape of the access cavity to the pulp chamber in an upper first premolar.

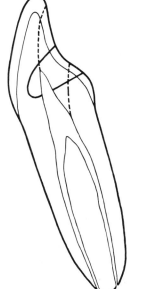

Fig. 14.9 Poor access (*solid line*) in a lower incisor can prevent a lingual canal being found unless its shape is altered (*dotted line*). Careless preparation can lead to gouging of the labial wall.

CANAL LENGTH

The length of the root canal must be determined so that preparation of the canal can be undertaken to the correct length. Otherwise if the preparation were too short, a ledge which could not be bypassed might be created, or if it were too long, the natural apical constriction would be overenlarged, making difficult the subsequent containment of the filling within the canal. From the preoperative paralleling technique radiograph, the approximate length of each canal can be assessed; this is a guide for the fine root canal file which is used for measurement.

A fine root canal file is inserted into the canal of the tooth to the estimated distance or slightly shorter if a stop is felt. The rubber marker on the instrument is adjusted to be level with a suitable reference point, such as the incisal edge. If the operator has access to an electronic apex locator, it may be used to verify the position of the file before a radiograph (bisecting angle technique) is taken with the rubber dam, clamp and frame all in position; the use of a nylon frame, being radiolucent, allows it to be kept in position. For a premolar

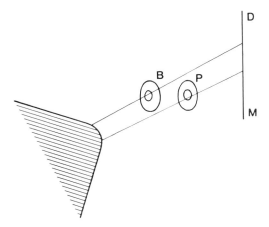

Fig. 14.10 When the X-ray beam is angled distally, the two root canals of an upper premolar appear separated on a radiograph; the buccal is the more distal.

tooth, instruments would be placed in each canal, and cusps or ridges used as reference points. For an upper premolar with two canals, the X-ray beam should be angled distally to separate the images of the canals; the buccal canal will be the more distal on the film (Fig. 14.10). The X-ray film is held in the mouth by the patient's thumb or finger and it is important that the film lies flat and is not bent, otherwise a distorted image would be produced.

The developed radiograph should indicate how close the tip of the instrument is to the apex (Fig. 14.11). The canal should be prepared to the apical constriction, which is approximately 1 mm short of the apex seen on the radiograph. If the tip of the instrument on the radiograph is within 3 mm of this position, the length is corrected and preparation of the canal performed without taking a further radiograph. Where the error is greater, the length is adjusted and a further radiograph taken to verify accuracy.

PREPARATION

The aims of preparation are to clean out the pulp and its remnants, and to shape the canal to allow the placement of the canal filling. This results in a flared preparation.

The canal is prepared with standardized files in strict sequence. A push–pull filing action is principally used to remove dentine. A smaller amount of turning action may be used in straight canals, but it is always limited to quarter-turns to prevent excessive gouging in the apical part of the canal. A turning action of files in curved canals should be avoided, otherwise it is very likely to distort the canal shape.

Fig. 14.11 Radiographs of root treatment in an upper premolar; *Left*: preoperative. *Left middle*: a file in the root canal for measurement of canal length. *Right middle*: after insertion of the root filling. *Right*: follow-up at 6 months shows the periapical lesion to have virtually disappeared.

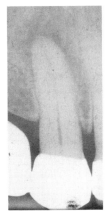
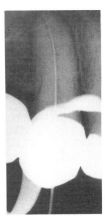
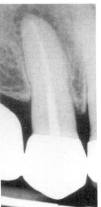
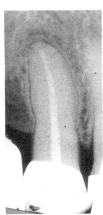

Many techniques have been recommended for preparing root canals; however, the one which is described is considered to achieve the objectives best, whilst minimizing the disadvantages. It is referred to as the step-down technique, and was described by Goerig *et al.* (1982). It can be divided into the following stages:

1 Coronal flare.
2 Apical preparation.
3 Stepback.
4 Final flare.

Coronal flare

The pulp chamber should be washed out with hypochlorite solution (see irrigation, page 204) and left flooded. A size 15 Hedstrom file is inserted to approximately three-quarters the length of the root canal, and then pulled back in a rasping action. The file is then reinserted and the filing repeated, working the file round the walls of the canal systematically until the file is loose. The orifice of the canal should then be irrigated slowly with a fine syringe. The filing action is repeated with the next sized file to the same or slightly shorter depth. This is then repeated with a size 25 file.

Apical preparation

A size 10 or 15 K-flex file is inserted to the full working length of the canal verified from the length radiograph, and then pulled back in a filing action. It is reinserted and the filing action repeated, working round the canal walls until the file is loose. The instrument should be removed from the canal frequently to allow cleaning of debris from the flutes with a piece of gauze and also for irrigation. Filing is then continued with the next sized file. Should it bind, more filing must be done with the last instrument. This sequence is repeated until a size 25 file easily fits to the working length; this is the usual size for a curved canal in a fully formed molar. In the canal of an upper incisor which has a fully formed root, it is normal to enlarge the preparation apically to size 40 or 50; however, in a young patient, the size could be much larger. As the instruments increase in size they become considerably stiffer. A size 25 file can follow the curvature of a canal whereas larger sizes, because of their stiffness, tend to straighten out the preparation of a curved canal. With curved canals it is usual to precurve the files.

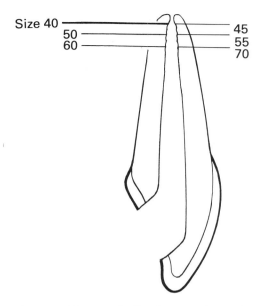

Size 40

50
60

45

55
70

Fig. 14.12 Diagram of a flared preparation ready for insertion of gutta-percha by the lateral condensation technique.

Stepback

After the apical part of the canal has been prepared to the appropriate size, the more coronal part of the canal is enlarged further, but as the size of each successive instrument increases, the length of preparation is decreased by 1 mm. This produces a flared preparation (Fig. 14.12). Between each size of instrument the canal is irrigated and the largest instrument which went to the full length is reinserted to remove debris compacted apically. Most root canals are oval in cross-section so it is important that the poles of the canals are filed with the largest size instrument which went to the full length, to smooth irregularities in the canal walls and remove debris.

Final flare

The coronal part of the canal is finally flared with Gates Glidden burs, starting with the smallest (size 1). The slowly rotating bur is introduced into the canal with minimal force to a maximum depth of three-quarters the canal length. It is followed by a size 2 bur to a shorter depth: in a molar, only the head of the bur should be inserted in the canal. The head of the size 3 bur would only be partially introduced into a molar canal; however, in an upper incisor larger burs could safely be used.

After this flaring the canal should be liberally irrigated, and the largest file used to the full length of the canal reinserted to rasp out any remaining debris. The file should also be used to smooth out any irregularities felt on the canal walls. At completion, the file should slide easily down any wall of the canal.

By carrying out the apical preparation after initial coronal filing, apical preparation is easier, the canal shape is likely to be better, there is less chance of forcing debris through the apical foramen and irrigation is improved. This method of root canal preparation is a modification of the stepback technique (Mullaney, 1979).

IRRIGATION

It is essential to wash out as much debris as possible from the root canal before and during preparation to prevent it from being compacted apically. Debris left in the canal may also act as a source of continuing irritation, and must therefore be removed. Frequent and profuse irrigation of the root canal is essential. The most widely used irrigating solution is sodium hypochlorite, in a strength between 1 and 5 per cent. It kills micro-organisms and dissolves pulp tissue, in addition to flushing out debris. To be effective it should be introduced far up into the canal and this requires use of an appropriately fine needle on the syringe. The irrigant must be syringed in slowly without pressure because it must not be forced through the apical foramen; if that were to happen the patient would experience an unpleasant reaction. During instrumentation of the root canal, the canal should be flooded with sodium hypochlorite.

The use of saline solutions for irrigation has now been discontinued because they are not bactericidal.

MEDICATION

After the canal has been prepared by filing and accompanying irrigation, it is ready for filling. However, this is not always done immediately, especially if there was periapical disease or, in the case of a vital pulp, the operator does not have sufficient time to carry on and fill the canal. Should filling be postponed to the subsequent visit, then the canal is dried with sterile paper points until they appear dry, before a medicament is introduced into the pulp chamber.

Formerly it was standard practice to place a medicament on a paper point in the root canal or on a cotton pledget in the pulp chamber. This is no longer done because many of the medicaments which have been used are now considered to be too toxic and a paper point could become jammed in the root canal. More recently, weaker medicaments, such as 1% aqueous parachlorphenol, have been used. Medication is no substitute for efficient cleaning of the canal and is not now widely practised in cases of vital pulp extirpation and because an antiseptic irrigant has been used. Nevertheless, it is advisable to use medicaments between appointments in canals which were infected prior to cleaning to prevent the remaining micro-organisms from proliferating. Leaving the canal space empty is not as effective as filling it with calcium hydroxide. A paste of calcium hydroxide with sterile water or a commercial preparation, such as Reogan (Vivadent, Liechtenstein), may be used as a dressing in canals which have been cleaned thoroughly, particularly if the interval between appointments is extended.

In cases of teeth with incompletely formed roots, a calcium hydroxide paste may be used to stimulate apical root closure, and in teeth displaying external resorption it is frequently used to control the resorption following thorough cleaning of the root canal. The calcium hydroxide should be used subsequent to thorough cleaning, not as a substitute for it. In none of these instances is the calcium hydroxide paste left as the permanent root filling.

TEMPORARY RESTORATION

After a medicament has been inserted, a dry pledget of cotton wool is placed over it in the pulp chamber before a temporary zinc oxide–eugenol cement filling is inserted in the access cavity; the temporary filling should be 3 mm thick and kept out of occlusal contact. Treatment is usually resumed 1 week later but should not be left for more than 1 month unless a calcium hydroxide dressing has been placed. Should the temporary filling give way, it is important that the patient returns immediately for canal cleaning and a new temporary restoration to prevent bacterial contamination of the canal.

FILLING

The root canal is filled to prevent the space becoming colonized by bacteria and being a source of irritation to the periapical tissues. The most widely used root canal filling is gutta-percha with a sealing cement. Gutta-percha has been used for over a century but no alternative has succeeded in displacing it. Silver points, which at one time seemed likely to displace gutta-percha as the material of choice, are not now used because they do not fit the canal well and are prone to corrosion, especially if the technique for using them is imperfect. The corrosion products may cause periapical inflammation and even discoloration of the mucous membrane overlying the apex.

The preparation of a flared canal facilitates canal filling with gutta-percha, particularly in the smaller sizes. A gutta-percha cone of the same nominal size as the last file which went to the full length of the canal is tried in the dried canal; it should fit snugly with slight resistance to withdrawal and it should be impossible to push the cone further apically when a spreader is inserted alongside. At this stage a radiograph (bisecting angle) should be taken with the gutta-percha cone in position. The developed radiograph should show the cone in, or 0.5 mm short of, the position to which the canal was prepared. However, it may be shorter if errors have occurred; it is necessary to check that the cone did not slip down the canal just prior to the radiograph being taken. If preparation has been carried out to the right length but the gutta-percha cone does not pass to the correct length, a slightly finer cone should be selected and tried in the canal. If the preparation is short it should be extended if possible. However, if the gutta-percha cone is too long and has passed into the periapical tissues, excess length should be trimmed from the apical end with a scalpel on a glass slab.

When a gutta-percha cone which fits snugly to the correct length is

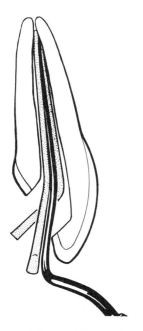

Fig. 14.13 Diagram of the canal being filled with gutta-percha; the chosen standardized cone fits snugly to the correct length. A fine root canal spreader is inserted alongside the cone to create space for an accessory point; this is repeated until the canal is filled.

found, the canal should be redried with paper points to prevent hastened setting of the root canal cement. A root canal sealing cement based on zinc oxide–eugenol cement is chosen (e.g. Tubli-seal, Kerr, Romulus, Michigan, USA) and mixed according to the manufacturer's directions. The sealing cement is usually composed of zinc oxide, with radiopaque salts such as barium sulphate added to increase radiopacity and natural resin added to improve the working properties of the cement.

The walls of the root canal should be coated with the cement, which has a thick creamy consistency, using a paper point dipped in the cement. The gutta-percha cone is coated with cement and inserted into the canal to the correct length. A fine root canal spreader is inserted alongside the cone and pushed, rotated and withdrawn to create space for a fine accessory point which is then inserted. The spreader is reinserted and the process repeated until the canal is filled (Fig. 14.13).

A radiograph should be taken to verify that the filling is adequate, neither underextended nor overextended and that the canal is completely filled (Fig. 14.11). If it is inadequate it should be removed and redone; slight overfilling, particularly of excess cement, is acceptable and should be left.

The excess gutta-percha protruding out of the access cavity should be removed with a heated instrument. A temporary restoration should be placed in the access cavity prior to definitive restoration of the tooth (Chapter 15).

14.6 Follow-up

Before the tooth is permanently restored after root canal treatment, the tooth should:
1 be free from pain;
2 show no evidence of tenderness, swelling or a sinus tract. Immediately after treatment there may be some slight discomfort but this should disappear within a few days.

The root-filled tooth should be re-examined after 6 months, 1 year and then annually for at least the next 2 years. The tooth should remain free from pain, tenderness and the presence of a swelling or a sinus tract. Paralleling technique radiographs should be taken to observe that a pre-existing periapical lesion becomes smaller and disappears, and that a new lesion does not develop. Following root canal treatment, periapical lesions which were visible radiographically should disappear within 2 years, although a few may take longer. If a lesion is still of some size after 2 years, it is unlikely to heal and root canal treatment may need to be redone or surgery considered. The majority of failures occur because of inadequate technique. Many operators have changed their filling technique from the single cone method to the lateral condensation method described, to ensure better filling of the root canal and so reduce failures.

There have been a number of studies over the years to review the success of treatment, which is in excess of 80 per cent.

14.7 Removal of old root fillings

Inadequate root fillings often need to be removed and replaced because they are associated with periapical disease. Before a root filling is replaced a preoperative radiograph should be taken to assess the condition of the tooth and of the periapical tissues, the material which has been used for root filling and the problems that are likely to be encountered. Often the existing root filling has been inadequately placed and does not fill the canal satisfactorily with regard to width and length. The tooth should be isolated and access gained to the pulp chamber.

If the existing root filling is a single gutta-percha cone, it is usually possible to work a K-file up the side and clear some of the root canal cement. A Hedstrom file may then be inserted and pulled out against the gutta-percha, which becomes dislodged. If the gutta-percha stubbornly resists removal, it may be dissolved with a solvent such as chloroform carried into the canal on the beaks of tweezers.

If the existing root filling is a full-length silver cone, it may be possible to grasp the protruding end in the pulp chamber with a pair of locking tweezers, or elevate it with an excavator.

If the existing filling is solely paste it is often possible to work through or alongside it with a K-file. The paste should then be washed out with copious irrigation.

If there is solely an apical filling of a silver cone or amalgam, its removal is difficult, if not impossible. Where treatment has failed because of a lateral canal coronal to the apical filling, resolution may follow the filling of the remainder of the canal with laterally condensed gutta-percha and sealer. In a very limited number of cases, surgical procedures may be necessary.

After the old root filling has been removed, canal length should be determined and treatment may proceed as described in Section 14.5. This chapter has given only a brief introduction to root canal treatment and the reader should refer to specific textbooks on endodontics for a much fuller description.

Bibliography

Goerig A. C., Michelich R. J. & Schultz H. H. (1982) Instrumentation of root canals in molar using the step-down technique. *Journal of Endodontics*, **8**, 550–554.

Gutmann J. L., Dumsha T. C. & Lovdahl P. E (1988) *Problem Solving in Endodontics. Prevention, Identification and Management*. Year Book, Chicago.

Harty F. J. (1990) *Endodontics in Clinical Practice*, 3rd edn. Wright, London.

Mullaney, T. P. (1979) Instrumentation of finely curved canals. *Dental Clinics of North America*, **23**, 575–592.

Stock C. J. R. & Nehammer C. F. (1990) *Endodontics in Practice*, 2nd edn. British Dental Association, London.

15 Restoration of pulpless teeth

15.1 Assessment

Before a root-filled tooth is restored, the quality of the root filling must be assessed, particularly as it may not have just been placed by the operator. If the root filling is inadequate it must be replaced before the tooth is restored, especially if it is planned to place a crown or if it would be impossible to replace the root filling at a later date because of the presence of a post in the root canal.

The crown of a tooth is weakened considerably by the removal of dentine to prepare an access cavity to the pulp. Remaining cusps of posterior teeth are prone to subsequent fracture, particularly if mesial or distal cavities are present as well. This gives the clinical impression that root-filled teeth are brittle, although there is conflicting scientific evidence that dentine is more brittle in a pulpless tooth.

Where the crown of an anterior tooth has not been weakened by caries, the access cavity may often be restored by a simple filling. However, where the mesial and distal walls of the tooth, particularly a posterior tooth, have been destroyed by caries, it is recommended that an extracoronal restoration is constructed to protect the weakened cusps and prevent subsequent fracture of the tooth extending subgingivally. Where little of the clinical crown of a tooth remains, a post crown should be constructed.

15.2 Intracoronal restorations

For most anterior teeth where the access cavity does not join any other restoration, a plastic restorative material may be used to fill the single surface cavity. The temporary restoration should be removed to a depth of 5 mm with a bur in the turbine handpiece, leaving some of the zinc oxide–eugenol cement as a base. A fine bevel should be placed around the cavity margin; however, the cavo-surface angle may already provide this incisally. The deeper part of the cavity should be restored with glass ionomer cement and then veneered with composite resin using acid-etched enamel for retention (page 138). If the surface is not exposed to wear from opposing teeth, glass ionomer cement may be used as the sole restorative material, in which case the cavity margins would not be bevelled.

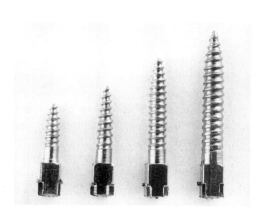

Fig. 15.1 A range of Dentatus screws for fitting into root canals to retain plastic restorative materials.

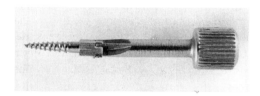

Fig. 15.2 A Dentatus screw and the holder used to insert it.

On a posterior tooth where there is no approximal cavity or restoration, the occlusal access cavity may simply be restored with amalgam unless the teeth show marked wear facets. However, if there were a pre-existing restoration involving one or both approximal surfaces, the tooth would ultimately be restored by an extracoronal restoration. As a preliminary, the mesial or distal remnants of the amalgam restoration should be removed because of the high risk that the various parts could subsequently disintegrate either before the extracoronal restoration is constructed or during preparation of the tooth for it. After the old amalgam restoration has been removed the support of the remaining cusps should be assessed. Where support is adequate, an amalgam core should be placed. However, if the cavity is non-retentive or the remaining cusps are inadequately supported, the tooth should be restored with amalgam using pin retention as a core for an extracoronal restoration.

Where a cusp is additionally missing, the root canal may be used for extra retention. Gutta-percha should be removed from the coronal 4–5 mm of the canal with a heated instrument before a Gates Glidden bur in a low-speed handpiece is used to shape the canal for the post. A tapered post (such as Dentatus, from A. B. Dentatus, Stockholm, Sweden; Figs 15.1 & 15.2) which just fits the canal passively should be chosen. It should be coated with luting cement (such as glass ionomer or zinc phosphate) and gently pushed into position; it should not be forced hard or screwed in because it might split the root. An alternative is to use a parallel-sided stainless steel post, e.g. Parapost (Whaledent International, New York, USA); it should be fitted into a hole prepared with a matching twist drill. After the cement has set; excess may be removed with a bur; the occlusal length of the post should be examined, and if the post is too long it should be trimmed with a diamond bur in the turbine handpiece so that the post will be covered by at least 2 mm of amalgam occlusally; the tooth is then restored with amalgam.

15.3 Extracoronal restorations

These are provided where it is considered that an intracoronal restoration would be insufficient, such as a posterior tooth with little remaining coronal dentine, loss of an approximal wall or a tooth with wear facets. With posterior teeth it is usually necessary to construct an amalgam core to allow the veneer crown to be of minimum thickness. Where buccal and lingual surfaces of the tooth remain intact, an onlay restoration is preferable to a complete veneer crown. These restorations have been considered in Chapters 11 and 12.

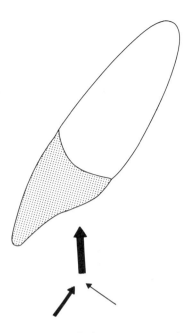

Fig. 15.3 Forces applied to a post crown have a lateral as well as a vertical component.

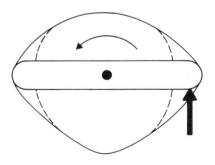

Fig. 15.4 A force applied to one incisal angle will attempt to rotate the post crown unless the shape of the preparation resists it.

15.4 Post crowns

A post crown is required to restore tooth where there is inadequate tooth substance remaining for a simple restoration or a veneer crown.

A post crown has a post which is fitted into the root canal and this provides retention for the coronal restoration, but it does not reinforce the root. It has become common practice to make a post with an integral coronal core over which a jacket crown can be made. This allows subsequent replacement of the jacket crown, on the grounds of appearance, to be made without disturbing the post. Whilst this is a simple concept and the ultimate restoration for a tooth, a number of these restorations do not give their intended service. In the majority of instances it is because of inadequate technique rather than defects in the materials or method.

Post crowns on anterior teeth are subject to oblique displacing forces, which inevitably have a lateral component (Fig. 15.3). These may be considered as:

1 A rocking force as might be applied to remove a garden fence post. A short post is at greater risk of dislodgement than a long post, and it is also more likely to split the root. The longer the restored crown on the tooth, the greater is the leverage. A restoration with a long post and a short restored crown is best at resisting this dislodging force.

2 A transverse force applied to only one incisal angle will attempt to rotate the post crown unless the shape of the prepared root has resistance to rotation either inherent from the original shape of the root canal or from an antirotational groove made by the operator (Fig. 15.4).

3 A hammering effect from repeated occlusal contacts, particularly if there is a premature occlusal contact in protrusion. As a pneumatic drill breaks up concrete, so a hammering effect can break up the cement lute that retains a post.

Posts may be retained by a cement lute or by a screw thread. Whilst the latter may be more retentive, the former normally provides adequate retention clinically and is considered less stressful on the remaining dentine. Luted posts may be tapered or parallel-sided; both are clinically adequate but the latter are more favoured. The post must have a good fit in the apical part of the prepared tooth. The core should also surround the post in the coronal part of the canal to give a good fit. The post may be wrought, preformed or cast; the first type are undoubtedly the strongest for their cross-section provided that a suitable alloy is chosen; the preformed post is usually fitted to a hole prepared with a matching size drill and therefore has an excellent fit but is frequently the most expensive; the cast post is adequate provided that it is of sufficient thickness coronally (minimum 1.5 mm)

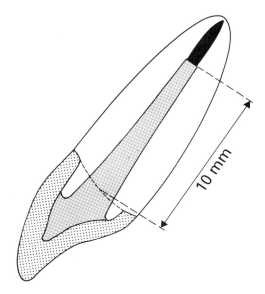

Fig. 15.5 The length of the post into the root measured from the approximal gingival margin of the preparation should normally be not less than 10 mm.

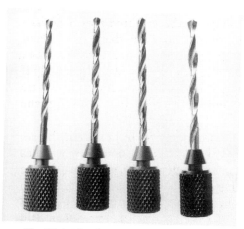

Fig. 15.6 The range of twist drills for preparing root canals. Diameters are (*left to right*) 1.15, 1.25, 1.35 and 1.55 mm. The handles are colour coded.

where it joins the core and that it is not porous. The post and core should be made of corrosion-resistant alloys.

A collar of coronal dentine should be retained where possible as it increases retention and resistance to displacement. The post hole should be prepared along the root canal approximately 10 mm apically from the approximal gingival margin of the crown (Fig. 15.5); the length may lie in the range 8–12 mm, depending on the length of the root. It is recommended that 5 mm of root filling is left undisturbed in the apical part of the root canal. Too long a post in the narrow apical part of the root may weaken it.

PREPARATION USING A WROUGHT POST

Preparation for a wrought post may be as follows:

1 The incisal half of the clinical crown should be removed with a fissure bur in the turbine handpiece. Filling material present in the pulp chamber should be removed to reveal the gutta-percha root filling. This is then removed with a heated instrument as far up the root canal as is possible, usually several millimetres.

2 Gutta-percha further up the canal may be removed using Gates-Glidden burs, starting with the smallest and working up to a size 3 or, in a tooth with a large root canal, a size 4. They should be used at low speed and their depth of penetration should be controlled by a marker on the shaft of the bur.

3 A hand-held 1.15 mm diameter twist drill is used to enlarge the canal. One dental manufacturer conveniently makes twist drills (Panadrills, Panadent, London) with small handles (Fig. 15.6). Gutta-percha is removed preferentially as it is softer than dentine. The chances of going off-course are considerably reduced compared with using an engine-driven drill. The preparation should normally be taken 10 mm apical to the approximal gingival margin of the final crown; it may be taken further provided that a 5 mm length of root filling remains.

The twist drill is followed by one of a larger size, 1.25 mm, which is taken to the same distance up the canal. Should the instrument bind apically the canal does not need to be enlarged further. If the drill is a loose fit, a larger size is used, 1.35 mm or even 1.55 mm. The size depends on the tooth, the age of the patient when the pulp died, the presence of caries and previous treatment.

4 The coronal end of the post hole should be flared with a long tapered diamond bur to eliminate any undercut inside the pulp chamber.

5 A shoulder for a jacket crown should be prepared.

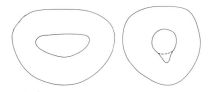

Fig. 15.7 Antirotational grooves. *Left*: the natural shape of the canal orifice provides resistance to rotation. *Right*: where the orifice is essentially round, a groove is placed palatally with a tapered fissure bur to a depth of 2 mm.

6   The coronal dentine is bevelled on the internal and external aspects (Fig. 15.5). If the canal orifice does not possess a shape that would resist rotation of the post, an antirotational groove should be placed in the palatal wall of the canal orifice with a tapered fissure bur in the low-speed handpiece to a depth of 2 mm (Fig. 15.7).

CONSTRUCTION OF DIRECT PATTERN CORE ON WROUGHT POST

A piece (approximately 50 mm long) of appropriately sized corrosion-resistant wire should be taken and its apical end smoothed with a sandpaper disc to eliminate sharp edges. Wiptam wire (nickel–cobalt–chromium alloy) has been widely used because of its strength, corrosion resistance and low cost. Iridio-platinum wire (90% Pt, 10% Ir) is an expensive alternative which has good strength and excellent corrosion resistance; platinized gold wire is yet another alternative. The strength and corrosion resistance of the wire used must not be affected by being heated to 700°C; for this reason stainless steel wire is unsuitable. The wire should be tried in the root canal and the part where the post will be covered by the core noted. The post is removed and fine shallow grooves are made in the surface of this part of the post with a carborundum disc in the low-speed handpiece. The wire is reinserted in the tooth to check the siting of the grooves, and to note the position where the post will emerge through the surface of the subsequent core. A deep groove is placed in the post around its entire circumference at

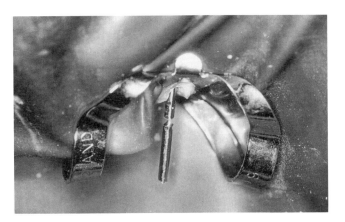

Fig. 15.8 The wrought wire post in the tooth with grooves prepared to retain the core and a deep groove where the excess wire will subsequently be separated from the post.

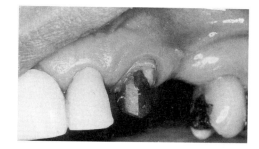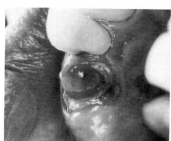

Fig. 15.9 *Left*: labial view of the finished acrylic resin core shaped in the form of a preparation for a jacket crown. *Right*: palatal view.

this position, leaving a central spindle of metal to enable the wire to be separated after the core has been made in acrylic resin (Fig. 15.8).

The post hole is coated with a separating fluid, i.e. microfilm. A small amount of Duralay acrylic resin is mixed to a fluid consistency. The resin is applied to the surface of the post except in the apical 5 mm. The post is inserted into the canal and, as it is seated, the resin should be carried into the coronal part of the post hole. Duralay is then built up around the post to form the core. When the resin has set, the protruding post may be pulled to remove both post and core, which is inspected. Should there be an air blow where the post fits the canal, further resin should be mixed and added, and the post reseated. When a satisfactory acrylic resin pattern has been obtained, the excess post may be rocked back and forth to break it off. The core is trimmed outside the mouth using sandpaper discs with frequent trial insertions to determine where excess needs to be removed. The core should be shaped in the form of a preparation for a jacket crown (Fig 15.9). The palatal surface must be trimmed to give adequate occlusal clearance for the subsequent jacket crown. If the post protrudes it may need to be trimmed with a carborundum disc.

After correct trimming the core should be removed (Fig 15.10) and taken to the laboratory for spruing on the labial aspect. The core is cast in a hard gold alloy, which flows around the post and locks in the retentive grooves; this is sometimes referred to as the cast-on technique. During the interval while the core is being cast it is normal practice to provide a temporary restoration for the patient.

TEMPORARY POST CROWN

The temporary restoration may be made from a plastic tooth-coloured resin with a wire post in the root canal for retention. An alginate impression of the tooth prior to crown preparation is used as a mould. A piece of cupro-nickel wire or stainless steel wire of similar size to

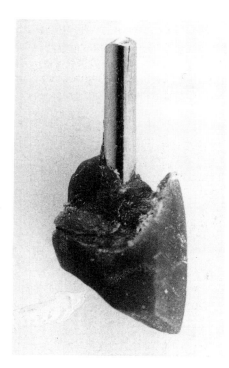

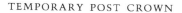

Fig. 15.10 The core on its post prior to being taken to the laboratory for investing and casting.

the permanent post is tried in the canal and grooved for attachment of the crown. Its coronal end is cut with wire cutters so that it terminates within the crown. The temporary crown material is mixed and inserted into the impression (Chapter 12, page 177); some of the material is coated over the post *in situ* before the impression is seated. When the material has set, the impression may be removed. The temporary crown is carefully eased off the tooth and trimmed as necessary. It is luted with temporary luting cement, which is usually adequate; however, in instances where there is no remaining coronal dentine, retention is reduced and it is advisable to fit the permanent post as soon as possible. Therefore, the interval between these appointments should be scheduled to be short, i.e. less than 1 week.

INSERTION OF POST AND CORE

At the subsequent visit the temporary crown is removed by placing a 2 mm wide chisel between the labial margin of the crown and the tooth, pushing it to the back of the shoulder and rotating. The preparation should be cleaned of temporary cement, with a twist drill being used to clear the canal. The post with cast core is then tried in (Fig. 15.11); the surface of the casting is left as a sand-blasted finish. The adequacy of fit and occlusal clearance should both be checked and adjusted; if previous stages have been carried out correctly it really should be ready for luting without further attention.

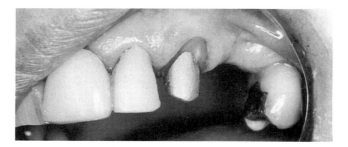

Fig. 15.11 The cast core tried in the tooth prior to being luted with cement.

After isolation of the tooth, the luting cement is mixed and applied to the post and base of the core; it is also well coated over the walls of the dried canal with a dental probe before the post is inserted. When the cement has set, excess should be removed, before the preparation for a jacket crown is refined, and an impression taken. The procedure then continues as for a porcelain jacket crown (page 182).

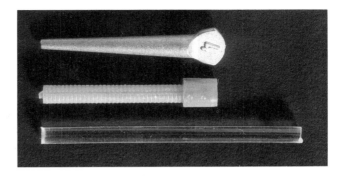

Fig. 15.12 Posts on which cores can be built. *Top to bottom*: a tapered metal post (Mooser), a parallel-sided acrylic rod with a grooved surface (Para-Post) and a parallel-sided acrylic rod with a smooth surface (Tical).

CAST POST AND CORE

A similar technique may be used to construct an all-in-one cast post and core. After the tooth has been prepared a parallel-sided acrylic resin rod, e.g. Tical (Palco, Colombes, France) or Parapost (Whaledent International, New York, USA) (Fig. 15.12), of suitable size is inserted into the post hole. At the coronal orifice of the post hole the diameter must not be less than 1.5 mm. The core is built up with Duralay and the procedure continued in an identical way to that using a wrought wire post. The post and core must be cast in an alloy which possesses suitable strength, such as a type IV gold alloy, and it may need to be heat hardened. After casting, an X-ray examination of the post and core should be carried out before it is tried in the tooth to ensure that there is no porosity.

PREFORMED POST AND CAST CORE

Should the operator prefer to use a preformed metal post such as Mooser (Precious Metal Techniques, London W1) (Fig. 15.12), an initial post hole is made with Gates Glidden burs to size 3 before using the manufacturer's engine-driven reamer in the low-speed handpiece; the size of the reamer is matched to the preformed post. The coronal end of the post hole must have a form that will resist rotation, either provided by the natural shape or by a deliberately placed antirotational groove. The coronal end of the post has a shape which will retain the core; this is built up with Duralay, as previously described for the wrought wire post, and trimmed. The pattern is invested and the core cast in gold alloy, which flows around the coronal end of the post. The post and core is tried in the tooth and when satisfactory is luted with cement before taking the impression for the jacket crown.

It is possible to construct the core in the laboratory instead of in the mouth, although it is not often advantageous. To do this, an impression is taken using a rubber impression material of the post protruding out of the prepared tooth. A model is made in the laboratory. The technician can then build the core in wax or Duralay around the post, invest and cast it. Because errors may occur in the alignment of the post, it is not recommended that construction of the jacket crown should be done at this stage; instead, the post and core should be fitted before a further impression is taken for the jacket crown in order to achieve a superior marginal fit.

Another method which the author does not advocate is to take an impression of the post hole in the root and make a cast post and core in the laboratory. This method has the greatest room for error in inexperienced hands.

PREFORMED POST AND COMPOSITE CORE

It has become popular in recent years to build up a composite resin core around a stainless steel post which has been cemented into the root canal, and then prepare the core for a jacket crown. Evidence to date suggests that this is an acceptable technique, which is quick to carry out.

The root canal space is prepared for a wrought parallel-sided stainless steel post, in a similar way to that for a wrought post and cast core (page 214). The post is then trimmed so that coronally it will finish within the core. It is luted into the canal with cement (such as zinc phosphate). After the cement has set excess is trimmed away in the pulp chamber. The root face should have a shape which resists rotation. The core is then built up incrementally with posterior composite resin and cured by light before it is trimmed with diamond burs in a turbine handpiece to conform to the shape for a jacket crown. It is recommended that the crown margins extend beyond those of the core. The core is finally smoothed with finishing diamond burs.

ERRORS

The following common errors may occur with post crowns:
1   The post hole may be too short.
2   The preparation of the post hole may have deviated from the root canal, thereby weakening the root and predisposing it to fracture.

3 The preparation of the post hole may have deviated from the root canal and as a result have perforated the root.

4 Preparation of the post hole may have dislodged an inadequate root filling.

5 The post may be too thin, particularly in the coronal part of the root canal, and as a result bend.

6 The post, if cast, may be porous and thus break.

7 An inadequate amount of luting cement may cover the post, considerably reducing retention.

8 Occlusal prematurities may lead to fracture of the porcelain jacket crown, remaining dentine core or the root.

In most instances it is possible to save the tooth but the crown must be remade; perforation of the root frequently results in loss of the tooth, although in some instances the defect may be successfully repaired; a fractured root inevitably means extraction of the tooth.

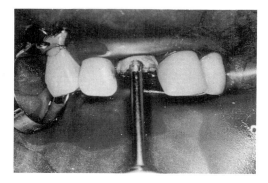 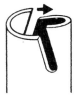

Fig. 15.13 *Left*: a Masserann sleeve being used to remove a post. *Right*: diagram of the cutting sleeve.

Removal of a post, should it be necessary, is best achieved by trimming the core until it is the size of the post and fitting over it an appropriately sized cutting sleeve of the Masserann system (Micro-Mega, Besançon, France). This is a plated steel tube with blades prepared in the end (Fig. 15.13) and it is held in a special handle which is rotated anticlockwise. The blade is intended to cut the cement lute. The cutting sleeve should be removed frequently so that debris can be cleaned from it and from out of the groove around the post. After most of the cement lute has been removed, the post suddenly comes away with the instrument. This method is less likely to result in fracture of the root than using patent post-pullers.

In the absence of a Masserann kit, the operator may be able to remove the cement lute from around a post with a small round bur

(ISO size 008) in the low-speed handpiece and vibrate out the post with an ultrasonic scaler tip. Particular care must be taken to remove as little dentine as possible with the bur to minimize weakening of the remaining root.

No post crown system is immune from failure; however, many failures can be attributed to inadequate technique.

Bibliography

Harty F. J. & Leggett L. J. (1972) A post crown technique using a nickel–cobalt–chromium post. *British Dental Journal*, **132**, 394–399.

Robbins J. W. (1990) Guidelines for the restoration of endodontically treated teeth. *Journal of the American Dental Association*, **120**, 558–566.

Shillingburg H. T. & Kessler J. C. (1982) *Restoration of the Endodontically Treated Tooth.* Quintessence, Chicago.

Sorensen J. A. & Martinoff J. T. (1985) Endodontically treated teeth as abutments. *Journal of Prosthetic Dentistry*, **53**, 631–636.

Stokes A. N. (1987) Post crowns: a review. *International Endodontic Journal*, **20**, 1–7.

16 Clinical environment

16.1 Position of operator and patient

Dentists suffered from backache for many years because of poor posture as a result of the patient being in an unsuitable position for treatment. However, in the 1960s a new approach to the treatment of patients emerged with the emphasis on the operator being in the best working position. This change was brought about by the increasing complexity of treatment and also economic pressures.

The operator is in the most suitable position when he is sitting down on a comfortable stool with feet on the floor and his thighs both parallel with the floor and supported by the stool. The seat of the stool should swivel easily and its base should be on castors which allow it to move readily across the floor. There should be a backrest to support the dentist's back, which should be kept straight while working.

With the operator comfortably in place, the patient's head can be brought to the best position, desk top height and level with the operator's elbow. This is achieved with a reclining dental chair which has a thin back to allow the operator's legs to fit underneath. The patient is positioned approximately horizontal with the feet at the same level as the head, both just higher than the waist.

The operator often works from behind the patient in the 11 o'clock position (Fig. 16.1) but may work in any position from 9 to 3 o'clock

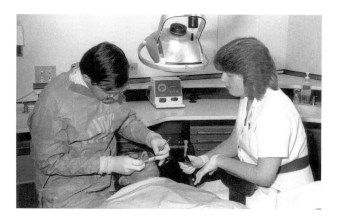

Fig. 16.1 The operator is on the patient's right side in the 11 o'clock position while the DSA assists from the 3 o'clock position on the left hand side.

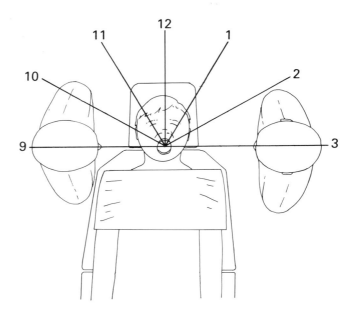

Fig. 16.2 Diagram of the clock positions. In this the operator is at 9 o'clock and the DSA at 3 o'clock.

(Fig 16.2). The right-handed operator usually works in the 9–12 o'clock zone, while the left-handed operator may prefer the 12–3 o'clock zone, provided that instrumentation is suitably positioned.

The DSA normally works in the 2–4 o'clock zone but would change sides if the operator chose to work in that position, particularly if he were left-handed. The DSA should have the seat of her stool higher than that of the operator to improve her view of the mouth. From this vantage point she can assist the dentist to make his work much easier.

It is helpful for treatment of upper molars to tilt the patient further back and so raise the patient's feet and, if the dental chair allows, tilt back the headrest.

The adjustment of the patient to the most suitable operating position is readily achieved with electrically operated chairs which often have preset programmes.

Although a small number of patients may dislike being treated in a horizontal position because they feel vulnerable, most patients find it very relaxing, which improves patient co-operation. Patients with severe respiratory problems may genuinely be unable to receive treatment in the horizontal position, as may those in the last trimester of pregnancy.

The use of an operating light is essential to provide adequate intra-oral illumination. Modern operating lights provide almost shadow-free light unless the operator's head gets directly in the way. The light should be approximately 1 metre from the mouth; for upper teeth the light is generally directed backwards and down, whereas for lower teeth it is usually more vertical. The dental surgery should be well lit to prevent the contrast between the well-lit operating field and the work surfaces from causing eyestrain.

All operative procedures should be performed with the operator seated; he should not stand to treat the patient.

16.2 Work simplification

The dental surgery should be designed to minimize unnecessary walking around. Equipment commonly used by the operator should be within easy reach and he should not need to stretch to pick up handpieces. Similarly the DSA should have aspirator tubes readily accessible as well as the instrument tray and a work surface for mixing materials. The foot control for the handpieces should be easily moved to suit the operator and be at his feet; it must also be simple to use. However, it should be impossible to activate it accidentally, such as by a castor of a stool. The turbine handpiece, low-speed handpiece and 3-in-1 syringe should fit positively into their holders, such that they cannot drop onto the floor, and they should have hoses which do not tangle. Handpieces should not operate until they are removed from their holders and the foot control activated; additional switches should not be required.

The operator should have a work tray close to the mouth for hand instruments. If he is working 'four handed' then the tray should be close to the DSA. A suitable work surface, on which materials can be mixed, and a cabinet of additional instruments which are used occasionally should be within easy reach of the DSA.

To work efficiently the operator should use as few instruments as possible. These should be arranged in a logical sequence in the work-tray before treatment starts. Burs should be selected beforehand and placed in a small rack. The laying out of unnecessary instruments and burs is confusing and results in needless repeated sterilization.

The exact contents of a worktray will depend on the procedure and the operator's personal preference. However, two examples are given.

A tray for examination should consist of:
mirror
right-angled probe
Briault probe

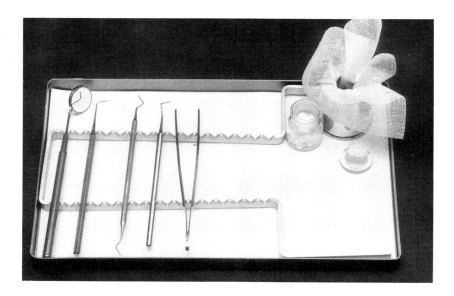

Fig. 16.3 A typical tray set up for examining a patient.

periodontal probe
college tweezers
pledgets of cotton wool
waste pot
and is shown in Fig. 16.3.

A tray for an occlusal amalgam restoration should consist of:
mirror
right-angled probe
college tweezers
front and rear binangled chisels
standard excavator
lining applicator
amalgam plugger
carver
piece of articulating paper
pledgets of cotton wool
waste pot
burs in rack:
    round diamond FG
    fissure diamond FG
    pear tungsten carbide FG
    round steel (012) RA
and is shown in Fig. 16.4.

The DSA can reduce the dentist's work considerably by carrying out many non-operative procedures. These are:

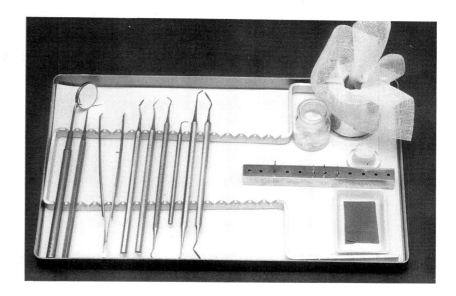

Fig. 16.4 A typical tray set up for an occlusal amalgam restoration.

1 Preparing the dental surgery before the patient arrives. The dental unit should be switched on and the supply of services, such as water, electricity, compressed air and suction, checked. The handpieces and 3-in-1 syringe should be tested for adequate function. The work surfaces should be cleaned and disinfected. The patient's notes should be taken from the filing system and given to the operator, along with any radiographs, and study models, and the worktray should be prepared with the necessary instruments.

2 The DSA should bring the patient from the waiting room to the surgery and seat him in the dental chair after outdoor clothing has been removed. A protective apron should be placed over the patient to prevent anything being spilled on his clothes. It is now common practice for the patient to wear spectacles (his own or some provided by the dentist) to prevent injury to the eyes by falling debris.

3 The DSA should place the patient in the appropriate operating position when requested by the dentist and adjust the operating light.

4 The DSA should pass the instruments to the operator for him to examine the patient's teeth. Instrument transfer should never be done over the patient's face in case an instrument is dropped. She should hold the instrument by its handle close to the working end so that she may place the handle straight into the operator's hand ready for immediate use. When he returns an instrument he should ensure that the DSA can conveniently and safely take hold of it.

5 The DSA should record details of the clinical examination on the patient's record chart as instructed.

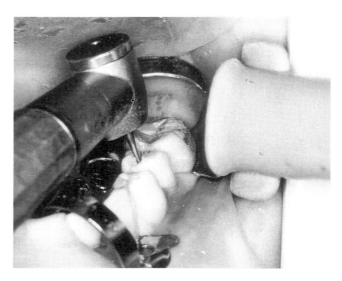

Fig. 16.5 The position of the aspirator during cavity preparation. In this example cavity preparation was carried out with rubber dam isolation.

6   The DSA should aspirate water from the mouth with the large bore aspirator during operative procedures. Because the operator is usually working from the right-hand side, the aspirator is positioned to the left of the tooth being prepared. The bevelled orifice of the aspirator is sited about 10 mm from the tooth (Fig. 16.5); it is not placed closer otherwise the high airflow would draw the waterspray off the bur. When a tooth on the left side is being prepared without rubber dam isolation, the aspirator acts as a cheek retractor. When a tooth in the lower right quadrant is being prepared, the aspirator acts as a tongue retractor. In addition, a high volume saliva ejector is often used to remove water from the fauces or floor of mouth. A competent DSA will ensure that she can see the effectiveness of the aspiration and give the best assistance without needing to be told by the operator. She may also use the 3-in-1 syringe to clear the operator's mirror, and to wash and dry the prepared tooth when the handpiece is removed.

7   During the restorative phase, the DSA should pass appropriate instruments and materials. In the case of lining material, she should place the applicator in the operator's hand and hold the pad with mixed material close to the patient's mouth. With amalgam she should place the material directly into the cavity if it is accessible or, where it is not, place the loaded carrier into the operator's hand. When a DSA

and operator regularly work together, she should be able to anticipate his next move and provide the right instrument; this allows rapid and efficient working. A practical guide to assisted operating has been produced by Paul (1972).

8   The DSA should remove excess amalgam from the mouth with a small bore high volume aspirator.

9   At the end of treatment the DSA should return the patient to the seated position and clean his face. She should arrange a further appointment and show the patient out of the surgery.

10   The DSA should clear up the surgery and sterilize the instruments.

16.3 Sterilization

Concern in recent years about blood-borne viruses has resulted in much greater emphasis being placed on cross-infection control in dental practice. Recommendations on appropriate procedures have been produced by the British Dental Association.

There are some dental instruments which will be inserted into the soft tissues and they must be sterile before use. Local anaesthetic needles come into this category. There is a much larger group which must be sterilized between patients to prevent cross-infection. There is a further range of equipment which does not lend itself to sterilization; at best, surfaces can be disinfected. Despite complete sterilization of dental equipment being impractical, the incidence of resulting infection is exceedingly small. However, this must not be used as an excuse for lowering standards.

Patients, who are the dentist's consumers, may well assess how good a dentist is by the cleanliness and hygiene of the dental surgery. There is, therefore, a need not only to practise good cross-infection control but to be seen to do so.

STERILE INSTRUMENTS

Local anaesthetic needles and cartridges must be sterile to prevent cross-infection. The use of disposable needles, sterilized in the factory by gamma radiation and packaged in sealed plastic sheaths, prevents the possibility of cross-infection. Similarly, the use of disposable glass cartridges of local anaesthetic solution, prepared and sterilized in the factory, maintains the chain of sterility. The accidental use of a local anaesthetic syringe on two consecutive patients must be prevented by a strict working regime of never loading a syringe until the time of actual use.

STERILIZED INSTRUMENTS

Dental hand instruments, such as mirrors, probes, chisels, excavators and scalers, and smaller items, such as matrix bands, their holders, root canal instruments and burs, should be cleaned and sterilized after use. It is most important to clean off plaque, blood, calculus, cement or carious dentine prior to sterilization because it hinders sterilization and looks repulsive when it is left caked on. Most detritus can be removed with a small brush and detergent, or by being placed in an ultrasonic bath.

The instruments should be sterilized in an autoclave. After wet sterilization, instruments should be allowed to dry to prevent corrosion, which can even occur with corrosion-resistant alloys.

Many older types of handpiece were unsuitable for autoclaving; however, manufacturers have recently produced handpieces suitable for autoclaving. The manufacturers' advice on sterilization should be followed.

The instruments should subsequently be stored in clean containers which have been disinfected; these may be instrument trays or drawers of a cabinet.

AUTOCLAVE

Most dental practices have changed from boiling water sterilizers to autoclaves in which high temperature steam, because it is under pressure, rapidly and completely sterilizes instruments. The sterilization takes 3 minutes at 134°C under a pressure of 30 lb per square inch. However, because the chamber needs to heat up and cool down, the sterilizing cycle takes approximately 15 minutes.

It is essential to ensure that the autoclave is approved for use and properly maintained since it is a pressure vessel which could blow up.

The instruments to be sterilized should be placed on a tray in the chamber, the base of which is covered with distilled water. The door must be closed tightly to prevent the subsequent escape of steam. The electricity supply is connected and the cycle start button pressed. The door cannot then be opened again until the end of the cycle because of its safety lock. The safety device is to prevent the escape of scalding steam and not to ensure that the contents are sterilized. Efficient sterilization may be verified by observing a change of colour on autoclave tape.

At the end of the cycle, the instruments should be removed from the autoclave and allowed to dry before being stored in clean containers for future use.

DRY HEAT STERILIZER

Dry heat is less effective at sterilization than wet heat so this method is slower than autoclaving and requires a higher sterilizing temperature. Normally, instruments and dressings are cooked at 160°C for 60 minutes; higher temperatures sterilize more quickly, but they also char dressings. This method is less widely used than autoclaving, is unsuitable for all instruments and, because the oven can be opened mid-cycle, may be subject to abuse.

DISINFECTED SURFACES

The operator's hands cannot be sterilized. However, they should be thoroughly cleaned with soap, and a scrubbing brush used to remove dirt from the nails. Patients like to see the operator wash his hands. It has become standard practice to wear rubber gloves. Any surface which the gloved hands then touch should either be sterile (e.g. instruments) or disinfected (e.g. work surfaces, switches and drawer handles). The operator should avoid putting his gloved hands on contaminated surfaces (e.g. his hair or telephone); if he does he should rewash his hands. This advice applies equally to the DSA.

The work surfaces, switches, aspirator hoses, tubes, bottles of materials and the handle of the operating light should be wiped over between patients with disinfectant. The spitoon must be washed down between patients and any debris removed from the safety trap. The aspirator hoses should be washed through between patients to remove debris which might cause an offensive odour.

Both operator and DSA should try to adopt an aseptic technique; where possible instruments should not be held by their working ends. During operative procedures the DSA should maintain a clean, tidy worktray and place dirty cotton pledgets in a waste container. Instruments which find their way to contaminated surfaces (e.g. the floor) should be set aside for resterilization.

16.4 History and clinical examination

It is very important not to rush into treatment. First it is necessary to take a history and follow it with a thorough clinical examination and any special investigations that may be indicated before devising a suitable treatment plan. Failure to do so could lead to avoidable mistakes. The history and examination must be undertaken to collect information about dental treatment in all its aspects, not just the restoration of teeth. Furthermore, the recording of the information is important as mistakes in doing so may lead to incorrect treatment. The clinical notes can become a valuable medico-legal document in cases where there is subsequent legal action, so the notes should be written clearly, completely and at the time.

DENTAL HISTORY

Before the patient arrives, the clinical notes should be read through if the patient has attended previously. The patient should be asked to sit down, usually in the dental chair, so that the history may be taken. The patient will be put at ease if this is done in a friendly manner. Considerably more is learnt if the patient is asked to describe things rather than the dentist interrupting to suggest answers.

REASON FOR ATTENDANCE

The dentist exists to treat the patient and not just to fill his teeth, so it is essential to know why the patient has come. There may be a number of reasons, such as the patient considers it is time that his mouth was examined, he may want advice or he may complain of a lost restoration, pain, an unpleasant taste, bleeding when brushing or unsatisfactory previous dentistry; the exact nature of any complaint should be noted.

PREVIOUS TREATMENT

It should be ascertained whether the patient is a regular or irregular attender, what is his attitude to diet, oral hygiene and treatment, and where and when he previously received treatment. If there has been a change of dentist, the reason should be obtained; the patient may have moved away from the district of the previous dentist, or he may have been dissatisfied with treatment. The operator should be wary of patients who change dentists frequently or for no apparent reason.

MEDICAL HISTORY

At the first appointment, the medical history should be checked in detail and updated as necessary at subsequent appointments. Whilst it is fortunate that very few medical conditions affect the provision of restorative dental procedures under local anaesthesia, it is necessary to know the medical conditions of the patient which would affect other forms of dental treatment, whether to avoid them or to take appropriate measures. The following should be asked:

1 *What is the name of your doctor, his address and telephone number? Are you currently under treatment?* It may be necessary to contact the doctor, particularly if the patient is under treatment.

2 *Are you in good health? If not, what is the problem?* The patient may admit to being under the care of a hospital specialist who is providing treatment rather than the general medical practitioner.

3 *Are you taking any medicines or pills, prescribed or not?* Some medication will immediately indicate the nature of the patient's illness, even if reference needs to be made to a directory of pharmaceutical preparations. Note should be made of self-prescribed preparations bought over the counter; for example, oral ulceration may follow the sucking of aspirin tablets.

4 *If you cut yourself, do you have any problems with bleeding?* If medical treatment is required following mild abrasions to the skin, surgical procedures such as extractions should not be undertaken without consulting the patient's haematologist.

5 *Do you have any problems with breathing?* Those who do will be unsuitable for outpatient general anaesthesia.

6 *Do you have any heart problems? Have you had rheumatic fever?* A history of rheumatic fever during childhood is usually sufficient to require antibiotic prophylaxis for procedures such as extraction and subgingival scaling to prevent a bacteraemia and possible endocarditis. Patients with myocardial damage should be treated in a way which minimizes stress because the damaged heart may be unable to cope with the resultant tachycardia and could fail; and electrosurgical procedures must not be performed on patients fitted with pacemakers because ventricular fibrillation could occur, with fatal consequences.

7 *Have you had jaundice or hepatitis?* Hepatitis caused by B virus is particularly relevant, and patients suspected of having been infected by it should be investigated by a suitable blood test. Because of the risks of contracting the disease from patients either with the disease or carrying the antigen, dental treatment is usually carried out under conditions of strict asepsis.

8 *Have you had any serious illnesses?* Epilepsy and diabetes are conditions where general anaesthesia is best avoided. Radiotherapy to the head and neck may cause a dry mouth and predispose the teeth to dental caries; in addition, tissues heal less well after radiotherapy.

9 *Have you been admitted to hospital?* The reason for such admissions should be determined. Most are of no relevance, except that they indicate that the patient was sufficiently healthy to recover. On the other hand, they may disclose facts which have not emerged so far, such as surgery to repair a cardiac defect which the patient regards as completely cured.

10 *Do you have any allergies?* Allergens should obviously be avoided. A number of patients are allergic to penicillin.

11 *Are you pregnant?* All women of child bearing age should be asked this. Whilst it is most unlikely that the radiation from dental radiographic procedures will harm the foetus, it would seem wise to reduce exposure to only those radiographs that are absolutely necessary, to avoid the first trimester and always to use a protective lead apron. General anaesthesia should be avoided.

12 *Have you come into contact with someone with AIDS?* This is a tactful way of approaching a delicate area. Patients who consider that they may be carrying HIV should be treated under conditions of strict asepsis. The number of HIV carriers continues to multiply and they are no longer restricted to a particular group of the population.

An alternative to asking these questions is to use a questionnaire and discuss with the patient those subjects to which positive answers have been given. Medical problems revealed by the history should obviously be investigated further by reference to a comprehensive text and to the patient's general medical practitioner or specialist. When the patient is a regular attender, periodic updating of the medical history is required.

CLINICAL EXAMINATION

Extraoral

This should commence with an assessment of the patient's fitness and colour before looking for facial asymmetry, swelling, sinus tract, ulcer or scar. It is unusual for such an abnormality to be present in patients who attend for regular dental treatment. When it is, the patient should be asked about its history and the abnormality should be palpated along with the cervical lymph nodes. If the patient has limited mandibular movement, an enquiry should be made into its history and the joints palpated during movement.

Intraoral

The mouth should be examined generally by taking a good look and by palpating the tissues. The lips, tongue, cheek, palate and mucosa overlying the alveolus should be assessed for normal appearance. The presence of swelling, sinus tract, ulceration or unusual colour should be noted. The teeth which are present and their excessive mobility as well as the presence of dentures should be recorded. A detailed examination of the teeth and supporting tissues should now be carried

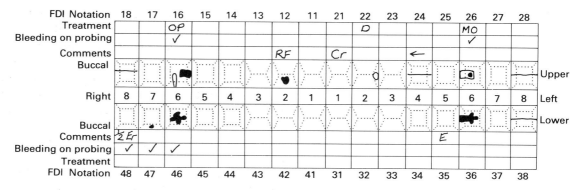

Fig. 16.6 An example of a chart on which details of the patient's teeth have been recorded. The symbols are explained in the text.

out. This is recorded on a chart such as Fig. 16.6 where tooth surfaces are indicated diagrammatically. A number of standard symbols are used to indicate the state of teeth. These are:

tooth absent	—
root present	+
tooth for extraction	/
cavity	O
sound restoration	●
unsound restoration	●O or ◉

In the box adjacent to the grid, comments can be made using abbreviations such as:

root filled	RF
crown	Cr
pontic	P
fissure sealed	FS
deciduous tooth	A, B, C, D, or E (or FDI notation)
tooth drifted	→
half-erupted	½ Er
mesio-angular	MA
horizontal	Hor
gingival recession	Rec
observe	Obs

In the next box, bleeding on probing the gingival sulcus should be recorded, usually at one site on selected teeth. Where there are several bleeding sites indicating disease, a fuller assessment should be made (Section 16.5). In the outer box, a note should be made of treatment required, such as:

distal	D
occlusal	Occ
occluso-palatal	OP
buccal cervical	BC
mesio-occlusal	MO
mesio-occluso-distal	MOD
pin	Pin
root filling	RF
fissure sealing	FS
crown	Cr
onlay	On

With increasing computerization, the FDI two-digit system of tooth notation is being more widely adopted, and this is shown outside the boxes in Fig. 16.6. For example, the upper left first molar is referred to as tooth 26.

The examination of individual tooth surfaces is performed in a good light, drying the tooth with cotton wool and taking a careful look. A mirror will be required for certain surfaces. Plaque should be removed with cotton wool so that the underlying surface can be properly examined. A probe may then be used to detect lack of surface integrity or deficiencies around the edge of restorations. The examination for caries has already been covered in Chapter 1 (page 13). Teeth appearing unduly dark should be noted, for their pulps may have receded, necrosed or been replaced by a root filling. The mouth should be examined for patterns of disease, such as areas of poor plaque control, erosion, cervical abrasion and areas with gingival carious lesions. This may allow interceptive advice to be given before definitive treatment is necessary.

Full details of diet and oral hygiene procedures should be obtained, particularly where there is evidence of caries, erosion or injurious or inadequate oral hygiene.

The vitality of the pulps of teeth which require operative treatment, those whose pulps are suspected of being non-vital or those with a history of recent trauma should be tested as described in Chapter 5 (page 54).

Where radiographs are required, these should be taken *after* the clinical examination. Indications for radiographs are given in Section 16.6 (page 242).

16.5 Periodontal health

Dental plaque, in addition to causing dental caries, also causes periodontal disease either in the limited form of gingivitis or the more destructive form of periodontitis.

The dentist has the responsibility to maintain oral health, not just to repair decayed teeth, therefore in the oral examination the supporting tissues of the teeth should be examined so that appropriate advice and treatment can be incorporated into the treatment plan.

If the periodontium is damaged, the support for the tooth is reduced and this may affect the prognosis of the tooth being restored; a considerable number of teeth in older patients are removed because of periodontal disease. The presence of plaque, calculus and gingival inflammation interferes with the restoration of teeth, so it is essential as the first phase of dental treatment to control disease of the periodontium.

THE HEALTHY PERIODONTIUM

The structure of the healthy periodontium is illustrated diagrammatically in Fig. 16.7.

The epithelium of the free gingiva extends to the amelo-cemental junction; superficially it is termed sulcular epithelium where it lines the gingival sulcus, while where it is attached to enamel it is termed junctional epithelium. The attached gingiva is bound down to the underlying bone and cementum by fibrous tissue, has a pale pink colour and is often stippled. In contrast the alveolar mucosa has a darker colour and is quite mobile. The width of the attached gingiva varies between patients and on its site in the mouth but is usually in the range 2–8 mm.

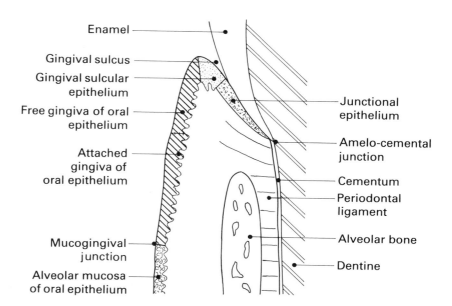

Fig. 16.7 Diagram of a longitudinal section through a healthy periodontium.

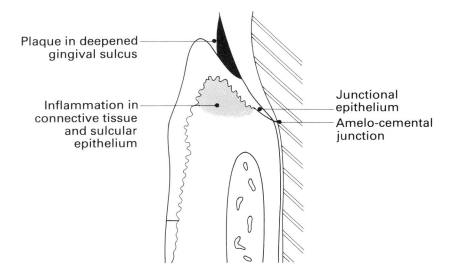

Plaque in deepened
gingival sulcus

Inflammation in
connective tissue
and sulcular
epithelium

Junctional
epithelium

Amelo-cemental
junction

Fig. 16.8 Diagram of a longitudinal section through a periodontium with established gingivitis.

GINGIVITIS

The structure of the periodontium in established gingivitis is shown diagrammatically in Fig. 16.8.

Accumulation of plaque on the tooth surface adjacent to the free gingiva causes an inflammatory response in the underlying connective tissue. There is increased blood flow in the gingival vessels, which may become visible at the gingival margin as well as causing a general redness of the gingival tissues. The gingival tissues are infiltrated with inflammatory cells and swollen, while the number of fibres binding down the gingiva is less than in health. The sulcular epithelium may be ulcerated causing spontaneous bleeding on probing. The apical termination of the junctional epithelium remains at the amelo-cemental junction. Plaque has grown into the gingival sulcus, which is deeper than in health. Initially the plaque is dominated by *Streptococci*, but with time *Actinomyces* increase and anaerobes, particularly *Veillonella*, become established. *Fusobacteria* and *Bacteroides* are present in small numbers.

With appropriate treatment gingivitis is regarded as being reversible back to health.

PERIODONTITIS

Gingivitis may progress causing destruction of the periodontal ligament; the structure of the periodontium in periodontitis is shown diagrammatically in Fig. 16.9.

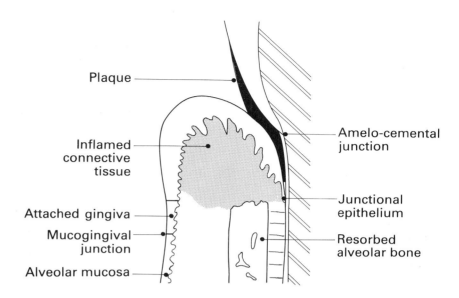

Plaque

Amelo-cemental junction

Inflamed connective tissue

Attached gingiva

Mucogingival junction

Alveolar mucosa

Junctional epithelium

Resorbed alveolar bone

Fig. 16.9 Diagram of a longitudinal section through a periodontium with established periodontitis.

The junctional epithelium has migrated onto the cementum of the root. The gingival sulcus has deepened to form a periodontal pocket. The surface of the tooth in the pocket is covered with plaque, which mainly consists of anaerobes such as *Bacteroides*, *Fusobacteria* and spirochaetes. The crest of the alveolar bone has also been resorbed. The extent to which periodontitis affects a tooth may vary from slight downgrowth of the apical limit of the junctional epithelium to exteriorization of one root of a multirooted tooth.

Periodontitis is not regarded as being reversible; however, with effective treatment further loss of supporting tissue may be prevented.

The transition from gingivitis to destruction of the periodontal ligament has been shown experimentally in animals but not in man. The rate of breakdown of the periodontal ligament appears to be cyclical, with short periods of rapid breakdown followed by long periods of quiescence. For most of the time there would appear to be a balance between the bacterial flora and the host response. In one mouth different teeth may be affected by periodontal disease in varying ways; therefore, it is necessary to examine the teeth individually.

CALCULUS

This hard deposit may be found on the surface of the tooth and is described according to its site. *Supragingival* calculus forms on the clinical crown of the tooth often close to the opening of a salivary gland duct, such as on the lingual surfaces of the lower incisor teeth. It has an off-white colour which darkens slightly with time and considerably with stains from cigarette smoke. *Subgingival* calculus is found in the gingival sulcus, or periodontal pocket; it is dark brown in colour and more tenacious than supragingival calculus. In addition subgingival calculus is more widely distributed in the mouth and the deposits are of smaller size. For many years calculus was considered to cause periodontal disease but, although it is calcified plaque, its harmful effects are due to the bacteria which grow on it.

PERIODONTAL EXAMINATION

The teeth should be examined for the presence of plaque on their surface; this is most readily achieved with disclosing solution and has already been mentioned in Chapter 2. Areas of particular plaque accumulation should be noted so that they may be brought to the patient's attention.

The presence and location of supragingival and subgingival calculus should be noted because these deposits will need to be removed *prior* to restoring the teeth.

The gingivae should be observed for colour, shape of papillae and texture. While healthy gingivae are pale pink in colour, have pointed interdental papillae and are often stippled, inflamed gingivae are red in colour, the papillae are usually swollen and blunted and stippling is absent. Gingivae which readily bleed are not healthy. Sites of gingival inflammation should be noted, for some surfaces of certain teeth may be more affected than others. A periodontal probe should be *gently* placed into the gingival sulcus to measure its depth at four sites on each tooth: mesially, buccally, distally and lingually. If the depth is less than 4 mm, it is regarded as clinically acceptable and not recorded. Pockets of greater depth should be recorded, usually on a separate periodontal examination chart.

If there is bleeding from the base of a pocket from *gentle* probing it is a sign of acute inflammation and should be noted.

The effectiveness of periodontal treatment will be measured by a reduction in pocket depths and the number of bleeding sites; therefore, an accurate initial record is essential.

The furcation of molar teeth may become involved in periodontal disease and therefore these sites must be examined. The loss of supporting tissue is often categorized:

1 Probe penetrates 1/3 width of tooth.
2 Probe penetrates 2/3 width of tooth.
3 Probe penetrates right through.

The mobility of periodontally involved teeth may be categorized:

1 Horizontal movement, 0.2–1.0 mm.
2 Horizontal movement, > 1.0 mm.
3 Vertical as well as horizontal movement.

Radiographs may be used to assess the marginal bone level, the presence of vertical bone loss and the presence of subgingival calculus on the approximal surfaces. When paralleling technique periapical radiographs are used, bone levels may be monitored to assess the effectiveness of treatment.

DIAGNOSIS

Many classifications of the extent of periodontal disease have been proposed; however, Lindhe (1984) has suggested that each tooth should be diagnosed separately and the diagnoses in Table 16.1. are based on his classification.

Table 16.1 Diagnosis of periodontal disease (after Lindhe, 1984).

Diagnosis	Condition
Gingivitis	No loss of periodontal ligament
Mild periodontitis	Loss of support < ⅓ root length
Severe periodontitis	Loss of support > ⅓ root length
Complicated periodontitis	Infrabony pocket, furcation involvement 2 or 3, or mobility 3

TREATMENT

This can be considered in five phases:.

1 Removal of plaque.
2 Removal of calculus.
3 Removal of overhanging restorations.
4 Removal of teeth in part or in total.
5 Surgery of soft tissue or bone.

Removal of plaque

Many patients admit to regular brushing of teeth but despite this fail to clean them properly. It is therefore necessary to explain the importance of effective cleaning, show the patient sites where cleaning is ineffective and also show him how to clean these areas better. Oral hygiene is the most important aspect of periodontal treatment; indeed all the other procedures are only carried out to facilitate oral hygiene.

Instruction in oral hygiene should consist of showing the patient areas of plaque accumulation after they have been stained with disclosing solution, before inviting the patient to remove the plaque with a toothbrush. This may make the patient realize how difficult it is to clean the teeth properly. If brushing is still ineffective or traumatic (i.e. horizontal), the patient should be shown a better technique of brushing. Co-operation is better where the patient is encouraged to modify his existing technique rather than being told that his existing technique is useless and that another is the only way. At the next visit the teeth should be redisclosed to assess the improvement. If there is no improvement the same advice must be given again, more forcefully, but still in a pleasant manner. However, if plaque levels are much reduced, it is then appropriate to move onto more sophisticated methods of plaque removal as the situation demands, such as the use of dental floss, toothpicks or special brushes. At each subsequent visit plaque levels should be reassessed to see that the improvement is maintained or improved.

Removal of calculus

Supragingival calculus should be removed to allow efficient oral hygiene. It may be achieved with hand instruments or an ultrasonic scaler. For long-term heavy deposits a short stout sickle, such as a jaquette, is very useful. Deposits on the concave lingual surfaces of lower incisors may be removed with a large excavator. Interdental deposits may be removed with a fine sickle scaler while calculus from wide (mesio-distally) interdental spaces may be chiselled off with a pushing motion from a watchspring scaler. The ultrasonic scaler removes supragingival calculus with considerably less effort for the operator; the instrument must be used with a waterspray to prevent the tooth overheating, improve the scaling action and prevent the handpiece overheating. While the ultrasonic scaler is being used, water should be removed from the mouth with a saliva ejector. Subgingival calculus should be removed with a fine sickle scaler, curette or periodontal hoe, depending on its site and accessibility. The ultrasonic scaler may also be used for removing subgingival calculus and has been shown to be as effective as hand instruments (Torafson *et al.*, 1979). The removal of large amounts of subgingival calculus from periodontal pockets is time-consuming but very necessary to halt periodontal disease.

Removal of overhanging restorations

Overhanging margins of restorations accumulate plaque, therefore overhangs should be prevented. However, when a patient is examined, an overhanging margin of a restoration placed by a previous operator may be discovered. If the overhang is accessible to trimming with a bur or stone then this should be carried out. Occasionally small thin excesses of restorative material (often amalgam) gingival to the main restoration may be pushed loose with a watchspring scaler and removed. Where an interproximal excess is not amenable to trimming, the restoration must be removed and replaced.

Removal of teeth in part or in total

Where a tooth has very little remaining periodontal attachment, it cannot be reinstated as a functional tooth and should therefore be extracted.

When one root of a molar tooth is involved with a deep infrabony pocket while the remaining root(s) is minimally involved, it may be possible to carry out root canal treatment on the sound root(s) and amputate the periodontally involved root. Such treatment would only be undertaken on a highly motivated patient.

Surgery of soft tissue or bone

This form of treatment is not now so widely practised because considerable improvement in periodontal health can occur with effective removal of calculus and self-administered oral hygiene procedures. The purpose of surgery is to expose the plaque-covered root surface which the patient cannot reach. Such a pocket would still bleed on probing after previous attempts to remove calculus and effective oral hygiene by the patient of the more superficial surfaces of the root of the tooth. Periodontal surgery is carried out some months after the inital phase of treatment — plaque and calculus removal. Periodontal surgery is contra-indicated in patients with inadequate supragingival plaque control.

INTERRELATIONSHIP OF RESTORATIONS AND THE PERIODONTIUM

A number of investigations have shown that restorations with subgingival margins cause greater gingival inflammation than unrestored teeth or restorations with supragingival margins, because of plaque accumulation. In addition, the gingival sulcus is deeper adjacent to restorations with subgingival margins. Therefore, whenever possible, the margins of restorations should not be taken to a subgingival position. Overhanging margins create more gingival inflammation (Leon, 1976), so these should be prevented or, if present, removed.

The presence of plaque and calculus on the tooth surface hinders the examination of teeth for caries, so these deposits should be cleaned off the tooth before examining the teeth for caries. The presence of plaque provokes gingival inflammation and bleeding on gentle probing; the bleeding hampers the examination of teeth and is a particular nuisance during operative procedures, such as tooth preparation, impression taking and insertion of restorative materials. Indeed, bleeding from an inflamed gingival margin can prevent an adequate impression of a preparation being taken. Gingival inflammation must be eliminated by effective plaque control before operative procedures are carried out.

When a tooth has been prepared to the gingival margin, it is important to check that the gingival margin of the preparation finishes on tooth substance and not calculus. If calculus is observed, it should be removed prior to impression taking, or prior to restoration in the case of plastic restorative materials.

The survival of a restored tooth is dependent on a healthy periodontium, therefore it is most important to maintain periodontal health. When treated periodontal tissues are adequately maintained, further loss of attachment can be prevented and restorations in these teeth can have a long life.

This description of the periodontal aspects of restorative dentistry is deliberately brief because the subject is very well covered in suitable texts, such as that by Lindhe (1984).

16.6 Radiographic examination

There are two main radiographic views used in the examination and treatment of diseases of teeth; these are the bitewing and the periapical. With both, the picture is taken with the film placed inside the mouth. Diagnosis can only be made from a good quality radiograph; this requires careful positioning of the film, correct angulation of the X-ray tube and careful processing of the film. A radiograph should be viewed against a uniform background light with the embossed convexity of the film towards the observer to ensure that it is not back to front.

BITEWING RADIOGRAPH

The bitewing radiograph normally shows the upper and lower cheek teeth on one side. Whilst the crowns of the first molar and second premolar are usually visible in full, those of the other molars and the first premolar are often only partially present; the amount is dependent on film position and tube angulation.

It is common practice to take left and right bitewing films on an annual basis for the detection of caries (Chapter 1, page 15) and for the assessment of restorations and marginal bone levels; subgingival calculus is also readily seen. In patients with a low incidence of disease, radiographic examinations may be less frequent. The apices of teeth are not visible on this film. However, it is possible to see whether or not teeth have root fillings present.

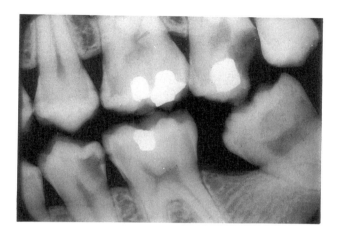

Fig. 16.10 A bitewing radiograph of the left posterior teeth; the radiological findings are described in the text.

A bitewing radiograph is shown in Fig. 16.10. It shows the teeth on the left side of the mouth. Teeth 25, 26, 27, 28, 35, 36 and 38 are present; both 24 and 34 are at the edge of the film and 37 is absent. Marginal bone levels are good and there is no calculus. There are mesial and distal carious lesions in enamel on 25 while 26 has a mesial carious lesion into dentine and two occlusal restorations. There is a very large distal cavity with possible pulpal involvement in 27 into which 28 has partly drifted. There is a large distal carious lesion well into dentine in 35 while 36 has a mesial carious lesion into dentine and an occlusal restoration in amalgam. There is occlusal caries in 38.

PERIAPICAL RADIOGRAPH

The periapical radiograph shows the tooth under investigation and often those adjacent. For many years the bisecting angle technique has been used (Fig. 16.11); this causes some distortion of the image, partic-

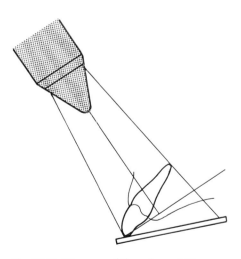

Fig. 16.11 Diagram of the tube and film positions in the bisecting angle technique. The central beam of X-rays is aimed at a plane that bisects the angle between tooth and film.

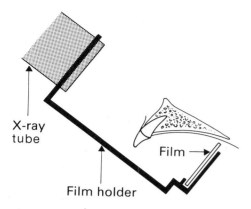

Fig. 16.12 Diagram of the film and tube positions in the paralleling technique; the film is held by the film holder and is usually some distance from the tooth.

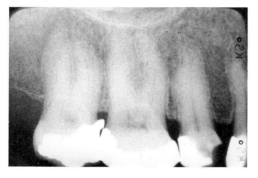

Fig. 16.13 A paralleling technique radiograph of the upper right posterior teeth; the radiological findings are described in the text.

ularly in the upper molar region. Because films are not taken at a standardized projection, quantitative analysis of information is not possible. The paralleling technique or long cone (Fig. 16.12) has now become more widespread because views are reproducible.

Periapical radiographs are normally only taken where there is a definite indication, such as:

1 to give some assessment of the pulp in a painful tooth;
2 to investigate the effects of previous pulp treatment;
3 to assess a tooth prior to root filling;
4 to assess a root filling;
5 to look for a root fracture;
6 to assess marginal bone levels;
7 to investigate the cause of a sinus tract;
8 to assess the periapical status of a tooth.

A standard size film is normally used for views of posterior teeth while a smaller film is used for anterior teeth. Figure 16.13 shows a paralleling technique periapical radiograph of tooth 16 which has an MOD restoration, no evidence of periapical bone loss and minimal loss of marginal bone. There is an MO restoration with a gingival overhang on 17, while 15 has an MOD restoration with the mesial part absent. At the top of the film, the floor of the antrum is visible.

PANORAMIC RADIOGRAPHY

Panoramic radiographs may look very impressive but the quality of the image is often inferior to that on good intraoral radiographs. Caries is better detected on bitewing radiographs and the periapical status of teeth, particularly uppers, may be assessed considerably better on a periapical radiograph. A panoramic radiograph enables the patient to be screened for unerupted teeth, root-filled teeth and a pathological condition of the jaws not necessarily associated with erupted teeth. The dose of radiation is approximately that of three bitewing films or 30% of 14 full-mouth periapical radiographs.

16.7 Treatment planning

The course of treatment must be tailored to the patient. An extensive and involved course of treatment is unsuited to a patient who has a neglected mouth and only attends for the relief of pain. However, in such a patient, a full oral examination is necessary so that the clinician can arrive at a correct diagnosis, can plan treatment properly should the patient be willing to have his mouth restored, and cannot be accused of incompetence or negligence.

Treatment can be grouped into the following sequence:
1 Relief of pain.
2 Control of disease.
3 Simple procedures.
4 Complex procedures.

The treatment plan which is initially formulated may well need modification in the light of events and it is always sensible to keep the plan simple.

At the first appointment, when the clinician examines the patient and carries out special investigations such as radiography and pulp testing, pain, if present, should be relieved; this will usually take the form of a temporary restoration because there is often insufficient time to place a permanent one, or removal of a pulp which is causing pain, or even drainage of an abscess.

It is common for the patient not to be in pain and attention may therefore be given straightaway to control disease. This will be dietary advice to prevent caries and guidance on oral hygiene procedures to control plaque. The amount and type of advice will vary from patient to patient, with some in need of extensive advice while others may need little. It should be given in a pleasant, helpful manner, as it is far more likely to be fruitful, and should be reinforced at subsequent appointments. If there is calculus on the teeth then this should be removed prior to restorative treatment.

Where a number of restorations are required, it builds the patient's confidence to start with a simple one which is accomplished without problem. Whilst it is attractive to carry out a number of restorations in one appointment, the patient should not be kept in the dental chair for an excessive length of time.

If during treatment the oral hygiene does not improve as expected, despite being reinforced at each visit, the treatment plan may need to be simplified. Similarly, if the patient is very apprehensive and difficult to treat, treatment should not be made unnecessarily long or complicated.

Complex procedures and those least necessary, such as crowns, bridges and dentures, should be performed last, only when the operator is satisfied that disease is controlled.

When it is intended to provide a denture for a partially edentulous patient, plaque control should be very good before construction is started. Further, the denture should be designed before teeth are restored so that restorations may be constructed with appropriate guide planes, rests and bulbosities.

When root canal treatment of a tooth is indicated, it should be carried out before the surface of the tooth, in which the access to the pulp will be prepared, is permanently restored. Furthermore, the provision of a permanent crown may be delayed to ensure that the root canal treatment has been successful.

Extraction of painful teeth which cannot be saved is usually arranged early in the course of treatment, whereas removal of symptomless teeth is left until later. After extraction, a socket should be allowed to heal for at least a month before restorations are carried out on neighbouring teeth, because the area may be uncomfortable and debris could fall into the socket.

The operator should try and make the most effective use of time to minimize the number of appointments and the total time spent in treatment, for his own benefit and that of the patient. This aspect is of considerable economic importance to the dental practitioner. The inexperienced operator will find that even the simplest procedures take a long time, but as he becomes more proficient they can be done more quickly.

It should be decided at the end of the appointment what treatment is planned for the next one so that a suitable amount of time will be allocated and any preparatory work will have been completed beforehand. The dental surgery should be ready by the time the patient is due, with the necessary instruments and materials prepared. The planned procedure should be carried out unless the patient presents with a more immediate problem, such as severe pain. While the operator is waiting for the local anaesthetic to take effect, he should be busy reinforcing dietary or oral hygiene advice, removing remaining traces of calculus or polishing a previous restoration.

16.8 Anaesthesia

Because of the sensitivity of dentine, most operative procedures are normally carried out on teeth with the help of local anaesthesia, which is simple to administer, safe and effective.

A small number of very apprehensive patients may be unable to accept treatment under local anaesthesia without the additional support of sedation; and for an even smaller group, general anaesthesia may be required for operative procedures. Details of sedation and general anaesthetic techniques will be found in an appropriate textbook, and will not be considered further.

There are some stoical patients who ask for, and happily accept, treatment without even local anaesthesia. However, most patients now expect local anaesthesia to be used for operative procedures on teeth. In restorative dentistry, a local anaesthetic is primarily given to prevent pain from dentine exposed during cavity preparation; subsidiary functions are to anaesthetize adjacent soft tissues, to reduce the discomfort of placing matrix bands or wedges and to reduce salivary flow and gagging reflexes.

The most widely used anaesthetic solution for dental procedures is 2% lignocaine with 1 in 80,000 adrenaline as vasoconstrictor. The vasoconstrictor prolongs the effectiveness of the anaesthetic by preventing its dispersion; without vasoconstrictor, the duration of anaesthesia would be unsatisfactory. The anaesthetic solution blocks neural conduction by interfering with ion exchange across the nerve membrane. Reported allergy to lignocaine is exceedingly rare and very few reports have been proven; and there is a wide safety margin between therapeutic and toxic doses. This is not the case with some other local anaesthetics, particularly procaine, which is now rarely used.

Local anaesthetic solutions for dentistry are usually supplied in sterile glass cartridges containing approximately 2 ml, depending on the manufacturer. These fit into special cartridge syringes to which are fitted disposable needles, 20 or 35 mm long (Fig. 16.14).

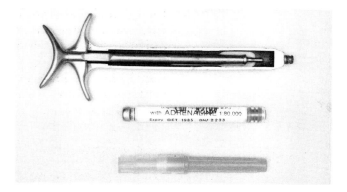

Fig. 16.14 A cartridge syringe for dental local anaesthesia together with a cartridge of local anaesthetic solution and a disposable needle in its protective sheath.

Most patients are apprehensive about being given an injection in the mouth. Therefore, the operator should reassure the patient that it is simple to do, virtually painless and totally safe. The operator's own confidence will allay any fears that the patient may have, whereas an unsure operator will pass on his insecurity to the patient. It is thus essential that the operator knows what he has to do.

The operator should be sitting comfortably with the patient lying in a position where the operator can see clearly. The injection site should be inspected and coated with surface anaesthetic solution or paste. This may be applied with a pledget or roll of cotton wool and allowed to act for approximately 1 minute; subsequent needle penetration is made virtually undetectable. Surface anaesthetics are effective on mucous membrane but not on skin. While waiting for surface anaesthesia, the syringe should be loaded with a cartridge of anaesthetic solution, which has preferably been warmed to approximately 37°C, and a suitable needle applied. The plunger should be depressed slightly to ensure patency of the needle and to eliminate air from the needle. The loading and checking of the syringe should be performed out of the patient's vision.

When surface anaesthesia has occurred, the DSA should pass the syringe to the operator and remove the protective needle cover.

The mucosa which is to be pierced by the needle should be carefully stretched by pulling on it with a finger or thumb. The syringe is then taken to the mouth, keeping it out of sight of the patient as far as possible. The needle is pushed through the stretched mucosa, while the operator distracts the patient's attention by talking about some subject of common interest unrelated to dentistry or by giving a reassuring commentary; the choice will depend on how anxious the patient is and how well the operator knows the patient. When the needle has been moved to the appropriate place, the plunger on the syringe is gently depressed and released to check that no blood enters the cartridge. After checking that the needle is not in a vessel, the plunger is gently depressed to inject the solution *slowly*. The initially injected solution anaesthetizes the tissues, making further injection of solution painless. Rapid injection of solution should be avoided as it causes discomfort. When the operator considers sufficient anaesthetic solution has been given, the syringe is removed smartly.

Prior to and immediately after the anaesthetic is given, the syringe must not be waved in front of the patient because it is likely to alarm him.

Sufficient analgesia for restorative procedures should develop within a few minutes. If it has not occurred within 5 minutes the injection should be repeated.

There are two types of injection used in the mouth: infiltration and inferior dental nerve block. The first causes anaesthesia by interfering with neural conduction in terminal fibres, and is routinely used to obtain pulpal analgesia in upper teeth. The second causes anaesthesia by interfering with neural conduction in a large nerve trunk; analgesia is produced in the area supplied by the nerve and its effect is more widespread than infiltration anaesthesia. The inferior dental nerve block is routinely used to obtain pulpal anaesthesia in lower teeth.

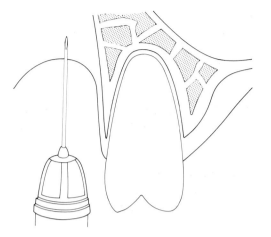

Fig. 16.15 Diagram of the position of the needle for infiltration anaesthesia of an upper premolar.

INFILTRATION

A single injection is given in the fold of the buccal mucous membrane next to the tooth to be treated. The adjacent teeth are also usually anaesthetized. On occasions when buccal infiltration fails to achieve pulpal analgesia, a palatal infiltration may also be given midway between the gingival margin and the midline of the palate, close to the root apex.

A short needle (20 mm long, 27 or 30 gauge) is normally used, and pushed through the mucosa 5–10 mm (Fig. 16.15). About 1–1.5 ml are injected to achieve effective analgesia routinely; lesser volumes are not consistently so effective. Greater volumes produce more profound analgesia without extending the duration of anaesthesia.

INFERIOR DENTAL BLOCK

The inferior dental nerve block is routinely used to obtain pulpal analgesia of lower teeth, because the thick cortical plates of bone reduce the effectiveness of infiltration anaesthesia. The inferior dental nerve block is a very reliable technique, and the use of less satisfactory infiltration anaesthesia is time-wasting and reduces patient confidence when it fails.

The inferior dental nerve block is not difficult although students often regard it as so through ignorance of the anatomy of the pterygo-mandibular space. The nerve is anaesthetized in the pterygo-mandibular space close to the foramen where it enters the medial aspect of the ascending ramus. The injection site is midway between the anterior and posterior borders of the ascending ramus at the level of the retro-molar fossa; in the dentate patient this is at the level of the mandibular occlusal plane (Fig. 16.16). If the retromolar fossa is palpated with the left thumb, there is a convenient depression to accommodate it, between internal and external oblique ridges of the coronoid process. The fingers may be placed extraorally to palpate the posterior border. If the lowest finger palpates the angle, the injection site is midway between thumb and third finger up. This technique is suitable for mandibles of all shapes.

A long needle (35 mm) is placed on the syringe. The needle pierces the mucosa just medial to the operator's thumbnail, and lateral to the pterygo-mandibular raphe, and passes through the buccinator muscle. The syringe should be aligned such that the barrel lies over the opposite premolar teeth. The syringe is advanced with the needle aiming for the midpoint of thumb and third finger up. Having entered about

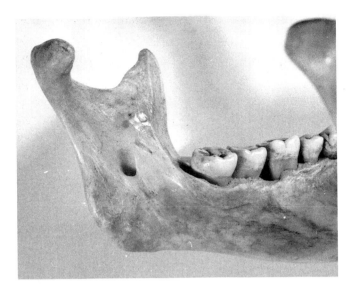

Fig. 16.16 The inferior dental nerve enters the medial aspect of the ascending ramus midway between anterior and posterior borders at approximately the level of the occlusal plane.

20 mm the needle should touch bone (Fig. 16.17). When it does, the solution is injected slowly until almost all the contents of the cartridge have been given. If the needle touches bone prematurely it should be withdrawn slightly and redirected a little more posteriorly. If the needle does not touch bone when inserted to 30 mm, it should be

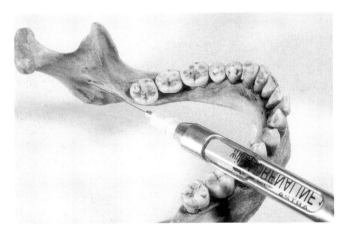

Fig. 16.17 The syringe in position for the inferior dental block.

withdrawn to 15 mm and the barrel moved to lie over the first molar on the opposite side and then advanced to touch bone. If the injection is given in the wrong site, anticipated anaesthesia will not occur. Injecting too far forward will cause anaesthesia of the lingual but not inferior dental nerve. Injection too far back may cause anaesthesia of the facial nerve in the parotid gland with consequent temporary facial palsy, or injection in the medial pterygoid muscle may cause stiffness on opening the jaw for a few days.

Because the inferior dental nerve supplies the lower lip, the adequacy of pulpal analgesia may be assessed from the state of the lip. The first sign of anaesthesia is a tingling sensation; as anaesthesia becomes more profound the affected tissue feels numb, swollen or even cold. To ask the patient to describe how his lip feels is far more revealing than saying 'does your mouth feel numb?', because the latter has the power of suggestion and is too vague. It should be remembered that the lingual nerve is usually anaesthetized at the same time but may be completely anaesthetized while the inferior dental nerve conducts nerve impulses normally.

The effects of anaesthesia last 2–3 hours and may be slightly longer with inferior dental nerve block injections. Following dental treatment, the patient should be advised to avoid eating, or biting the anaesthetized tissue, until the effects of the anaesthetic have passed off.

CONTRA-INDICATIONS

There are fortunately few contra-indications to local anaesthesia:

1 It is unwise to inject into infected tissues in case infection is spread. This is overcome by injecting away from or around the affected area.

2 Patients with severe bleeding disorders, such as haemophiliacs or those taking anticoagulants, should not be given injections of local anaesthetic without making arrangements with the patient's haematologist.

The often stated contra-indication that patients with cardiovascular disease should not be given local anaesthetics with adrenaline is unfounded (Cawson et al., 1983). The amount of adrenaline in a cartridge of local anaesthetic is insignificant with what the adrenal glands can produce when stimulated. It is most important to prevent stress in these patients by carrying out treatment in a calm manner and using an effective local anaesthetic solution; plain lignocaine is not nearly so effective because of the lack of vasoconstrictor. Prilocaine with vasoconstrictor is sometimes recommended as an alternative but its shorter duration of infiltration anaesthesia can be a drawback to the student operator. There is no clinical evidence of interaction between the vasoconstrictor in local anaesthetics and antidepressant medication prescribed to some patients.

COMPLICATIONS

1   If the anaesthetic is ineffective, a further injection should be given. Was too little given in the wrong place?

2   The anaesthetic may be accidentally introduced into a vein, although this is clinically uncommon. Whilst it is desirable to aspirate prior to injection, few operators do; several studies have shown that aspiration of blood into the syringe is more common than the clinical effects. Bishop (1983) in a study of children found a positive aspiration rate of 15%, which is about twice as high as previous reports. Intravenous injection may be followed by tachycardia, which can alarm the patient. Some words of reassurance to the patient can help to prevent the adrenal glands from prolonging the transitory tachycardia. The operator can be virtually certain that the injection will not have anaesthetized the intended nerve, so a further injection is necessary.

3   Occasionally, in giving an inferior dental nerve block, the operator scores 'a bull's eye': the nerve bundle is hit by the needle. This causes an unpleasant shock in the area of the nerve distribution but is usually followed by profound anaesthesia of normal duration. There are rarely more serious consequences.

4   On rare occasions, the local anaesthetic needle causes bleeding into the tissues from a small vessel to form a pool of blood, a haematoma. In many instances these resolve without treatment. With a large haematoma there is the possibility of infection, and antibiotics may therefore be prescribed as a prophylactic measure. The incidence of this complication has been reduced with the widespread use of disposable needles, which are very sharp and unlikely to tear the tissues.

5   If anaesthetic solution is injected into the parotid gland, anaesthesia of the facial nerve may result, with a temporary facial palsy. Muscle tone returns to normal when the anaesthetic wears off. If the eyelid is affected the eye should be covered for the duration of anaesthesia.

6   Fainting used to be a complication of giving local anaesthetic injections when patients were in the sitting position for treatment. With the patient lying down, fainting cannot occur because cerebral blood flow is assured.

7   Breakage of needles was a recognized hazard when reusable needles were widely used. It is almost unheard of with disposable needles. However, it is still advisable never to insert a needle right up to the

hub, where it is weakest, so that it may be retrieved with artery forceps should it break.

8 It is rare for a needle track infection to follow when sterile disposable needles have been used. It is essential that the operator and DSA do not touch the needle prior to injection.

Cartridges and needles for local anaesthesia are sterile when supplied and intended for one patient use only. This prevents cross-infection, particularly of hepatitis B virus, and ensures that needles are always sharp.

After use, the needle should be replaced in its protective sheath and disposed into a safe 'sharps' container together with the glass cartridge of remaining anaesthetic solution. It is the dentist's responsibility to ensure that the sharps container is not a hazard to surgery or cleaning staff.

16.9 Moisture control

It is essential when placing a restoration to avoid moisture contamination of the restorative material because its properties would be adversely affected; with some materials these adverse effects are marked, and also etched enamel can cease to be an effective surface for the bonding of resins if salivary contamination occurs.

There are two methods of preventing moisture contamination: rubber dam and cotton wool rolls.

RUBBER DAM

This is the most effective method of isolating teeth but it is not always the easiest. Therefore, many inexperienced operators avoid its use and never become proficient with it.

Rubber dam is a sheet of rubber, usually 150 mm square, in which holes are punched to allow the tooth being treated, and often several adjacent ones, to protrude through, thereby isolating these teeth from the rest of the mouth.

A proficient operator should be able to place a rubber dam within 1 minute and thereafter have a dry field. Those who routinely use rubber dam prefer to carry out the entire procedure, including cavity preparation, under rubber dam isolation because the working environment is saliva-free. The tongue and cheeks are excluded and the patient cannot put his tongue in the cavity when the operator is not looking.

It is most important to ensure that the rubber dam is effectively anchored to the teeth; therefore, a clamp which grips a tooth at its neck is routinely employed, particularly when molar teeth are isolated.

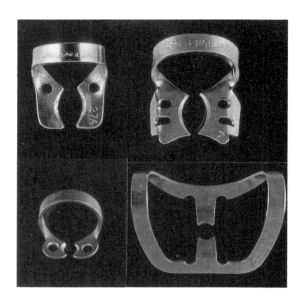

Fig. 16.18 *Top left*: a wingless molar clamp. *Top right*: a winged molar clamp. *Bottom left*: a wingless anterior clamp. *Bottom right*: a double bow wingless anterior clamp.

When a posterior tooth is being treated, the clamp should be placed on the tooth behind and it is usual to isolate several teeth (four or more but not less than three) in the quadrant to increase stability.

There are three basic types of clamp (Fig. 16.18): wingless, winged and double bow. The first two in various sizes will fit any tooth and they differ according to the method of rubber dam application, while the double bow clamp can be used on any anterior tooth. Clamps are placed on and taken off teeth with special forceps. Because anchorage is dependent on the clamp, the operator should first select a suitable clamp and try it on the anchor tooth to test its stability. If it is unstable, another clamp should be chosen. A winged clamp is placed in the rubber dam forceps, taken to the mouth and fitted over the anchor tooth. When it is in position the forceps are removed and the bow of the clamp is manipulated to test stability; it should not move. The suitable clamp is removed with forceps.

A sheet of good quality rubber dam is taken and placed on the frame. A punch is used to make holes for the number of teeth to be isolated, each hole approximately 10 mm apart. The clamp is fitted into the appropriate hole in the dam and kept in place by the wings of the clamp.

The forceps should engage the clamp, which is then placed over the distal tooth to be clamped, with dam and frame attached. The frame prevents the patient having an unpleasant mouthful of rubber. When the clamp is in position the forceps should be removed, and the dam is slipped off the wings of the clamp with a blunt instrument, such as a periodontal probe or flat plastic, to ensure a tight seal around the tooth.

The septa of rubber dam then need to be slipped through the approximal contacts; this is facilitated with a lubricant soap. The operator holds the dam on the buccal and lingual sides and positions the septum over the contact to slide it through on its edge. If the edge of the septum is not presented to the contact, the rubber dam bunches up and refuses to pass. Dental floss or tape may be used to pass the dam through difficult contacts, by working through one edge of the dam. If floss is placed on the middle of the septum, the rubber dam bunches and will not pass through the tight contact.

When the rubber dam has been passed through the contacts, the edge of rubber around the tooth to be treated often needs to be tucked into the gingival sulcus; approximally dental floss may be used, while buccally a blunt instrument, such as a flat plastic or periodontal probe, is most suitable. A wooden wedge should be placed between the rubber dam and the approximal contact where a cavity is to be prepared; the wedge retracts the gingiva and protects the dam from damage by burs during cavity preparation. Anteriorly another clamp may also be used (Fig. 16.19).

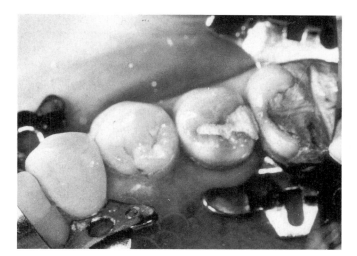

Fig. 16.19 Teeth isolated by rubber dam held in place by clamps; a wedge may be placed to retract the rubber dam and the gingival papilla where a cavity is to be prepared.

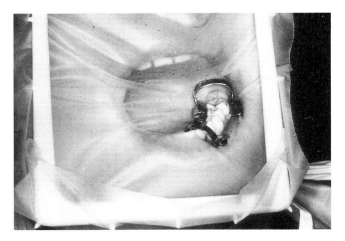

Fig. 16.20 The rubber dam has been turned over the edge of the frame to form a gutter which prevents water running onto the patient.

The frame should be adjusted if required and a napkin placed between the dam and face to make the patient more comfortable. To prevent water running off the dam, the edge should be turned over the frame to form a gutter (Fig. 16.20).

With the rubber dam in place, it is not necessary to place a saliva ejector in the mouth as the patient can swallow without difficulty.

When treatment is complete, the rubber dam is easily taken off. The clamp is removed, together with any wedges, before the dam is pulled through the contacts. Where difficulty is encountered or a restoration has been newly inserted, the septa should be cut with scissors, taking care not to cut the patient's lip.

All clamps should be applied carefully to teeth and the jaws must not trap the gingivae. Where the jaws are close to the gingival margin, it is more comfortable for the patient if the gingivae have been anaesthetized; for upper teeth this would require palatal infiltration of local anaesthetic.

With any procedure, but particularly with the application of rubber dam, as the patient may be unfamiliar with it, its purpose should be explained to the patient and reassurance given, particularly at the time of application.

An alternative method of rubber dam application is to place a clamp onto the tooth and apply the rubber dam over it *in situ*. This technique is valuable where clamp position is critical; a wingless clamp is normally used, because rubber dam can be stretched over it more easily than over a winged clamp.

For the treatment of anterior teeth, the rubber dam usually isolates the incisors and canines. Where contacts are tight and the crowns of teeth long, a strip of excess rubber dam or a wooden wedge may be used to wedge the distal contact instead of a clamp. If the operator considers anchorage might be insufficient, a clamp is used on the most posterior tooth isolated in one or both quadrants. A wooden wedge is used to keep the dam in place approximally on the tooth being treated. When a gingival cavity is being treated, a double bow clamp is often used to achieve sufficient gingival retraction of the dam.

Rubber dam isolation is necessary for root canal treatment to prevent salivary contamination and inhalation or ingestion of instruments. Frequently, single tooth isolation is used with a clamp placed on the tooth being treated.

There will only be a small number of instances when rubber dam isolation will be impossible, usually because the operator does not have a suitable clamp. It is possible to modify clamps for individual teeth (Elderton, 1971).

COTTON WOOL ROLLS

The use of cotton wool rolls and a saliva ejector is a less satisfactory method of moisture control, although it is widely used while a restoration is being inserted. The roll is placed in the buccal sulcus adjacent to the tooth, with a rolling action away from the alveolus so that it is retained by the natural elasticity of the tissues. If it were done in reverse, the roll would ride out. When a tooth is being treated in the lower arch, a roll is also inserted in the lingual sulcus. A saliva ejector is always placed as well, to maintain a dry tooth. If the patient is a profuse salivator, rolls may need to be replaced during the course of treatment.

16.10 Occlusion

Occlusion can simply be defined as any contact between teeth of opposing arches, although a great deal more is often implied. The importance of occlusion in clinical dentistry is to ensure that restorations do not adversely alter tooth contacts. No engineer would fill the teeth of a gear wheel to an indifferent contour with a dissimilar material, but that is what often occurs in dental treatment.

When the mandible is closed such that the opposing teeth interdigitate maximally, it is in the intercuspal position; the teeth are in *intercuspal occlusion*, previously called *centric occlusion*. Most

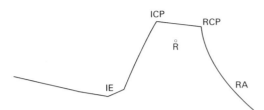

Fig. 16.21 The relative positions in a vertical plane of the incisal edge of a lower incisor tooth in different positions of the mandible. IE = incisal edge of upper incisor; ICP = intercuspal position; RCP = retruded contact position; R = rest position; RA = retruded axis where the condyle is rotated in its uppermost position.

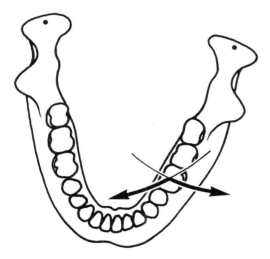

Fig. 16.22 In left lateral movement the mandible essentially rotates around the axis of the left condyle; the lower left molar therefore moves laterally. In right lateral movement there is rotation around the right condyle; the lower left molar moves forwards and to the right as the left condyle moves forwards.

patients can readily close into this position. *Normal occlusion* implies an ideal relationship of upper and lower teeth in intercuspal occlusion; a significant number of patients do not have 'normal occlusion', with little noticeable ill-effect.

When the mandible is in the intercuspal position the condyles are frequently not as far up and back in their fossae as they can be positioned. The difference in positions is of the order of 1 mm in most patients. The position of the mandible when its condyles are fully seated in their fossae is known as the *retruded contact position* (previously called *centric relation*); this position is not normally used in the treatment of dentate patients unless extensive restorative work is being carried out; however, it is used as a reference point in edentulous patients. The relative positions in the vertical plane for a lower incisor are shown in Fig. 16.21.

From the intercuspal position the mandible may be protruded or moved laterally; these movements are limited by the condyles and the articular surfaces of the teeth. In chewing, the mandible moves from an eccentric position into the intercuspal position. Protrusion is limited by the palatal surfaces of the upper incisors (incisal guidance) and the condylar path. Lateral movement is essentially a rotation around the axis of the condyle on the side to which the mandible has moved while the other condyle has come down and forward from the glenoid fossa (Fig. 16.22). The side on which the mandible has rotated is known as the working side, while the other is the non-working side. Often the only teeth that can contact on the working side are the canines, hence the term 'canine guided occlusion'. An alternative tooth relationship is 'group function', where several teeth can contact on the working side. There is not normally any contact between teeth on the non-working side; this is in contrast to the occlusion on complete dentures where cross-arch balancing contacts are introduced to create stability of the dentures.

During chewing, the masticatory musculature normally moves the mandibular teeth closely across the maxillary teeth but out of contact. Since opposing teeth rarely contact, wear is minimized. Excessive wear is usually the result of a grinding habit: parafunction. Loss of tooth substance by erosion can also destroy the intercuspal occlusion, leading to a new position of intercuspal occlusion with the mandible having slid forward or sideways from the original position.

Restorative procedures on individual teeth may interfere with the natural occlusion. If a restoration on the occlusal surface is overbuilt, it will cause a *premature contact* preventing closure into intercuspal occlusion. If the cusps of a restoration are made too large, they may interfere with mandibular movements. When a restoration is under-built without occlusal contacts, over-eruption may occur with the potential development of interferences in mandibular movement. These abnormalities of occlusion will be considered in turn.

PREMATURE CONTACT

This may be created by failing to contour a restoration correctly.

Premature contact on a newly inserted amalgam restoration may lead to part breaking off the restoration. Repeated premature contact on the tooth will make it sore and painful within hours; the periodontal ligament becomes inflamed causing extrusion of the tooth from its socket, thus increasing the prematurity. The tooth is likely to be hypersensitive to cold.

Should the patient return the day after treatment complaining of pain on biting, the excess restorative material should be removed to eliminate the prematurity.

In the absence of the prematurity being adjusted, the condition will gradually resolve with apical repositioning of the tooth. The long-term effects are likely to be minimal, particularly if the error was small. However, a greater error may cause pulpal necrosis, by obstructing blood flow in the vessels passing through the apical foramen.

The operator should have prevented the occlusal prematurity by contouring the restoration correctly at the time of treatment. Prior to restoration of the tooth, the patient's occlusion should be examined to assess the degree of interdigitation of the teeth and the positions of tooth contact in the intercuspal position using articulating paper. If interdigitation is excessive, as may occur if an opposing cusp has over-erupted into a cavity, it would be beneficial to reduce or round the sharp point of the opposing cusp to provide more room for the restoration and to reduce stress.

When the restoration has been inserted, the patient should be instructed to close his teeth gently together in the intercuspal position to observe the degree of tooth separation (i.e. the amount of excess material) and the positions of premature contact. If the contacts are not readily visible, articulating paper may be used to indicate them. The restoration should be adjusted until all prematurities in the intercuspal position have been eliminated. When there is a large prematurity, the patient is aware of occlusal contact solely on that tooth; as it is reduced, the patient will become aware of tooth contacts on the other side of the mouth. When the prematurity is finally eliminated the patient suddenly ceases to be aware of it.

The operator will find it far easier to insert one restoration at a time because only one tooth can cause a prematurity.

PREMATURITY IN FUNCTIONAL MOVEMENT

This is a more insidious contact because its presence is not immediately apparent to the patient. It usually occurs in lateral movements and may be created by overbuilding the cusps or ridges of a restoration. It is more likely to be created in a group function occlusion, because there is less room to accommodate errors than in a canine guided occlusion.

The interference may damage the restoration by fracturing part of it if it has been constructed from a brittle material. However, if the restoration is tough, it may become dislodged from the tooth if retention is poor, or the supporting core may fracture. Alternatively, the interference may initiate an abnormal grinding habit, which may lead to muscle spasm and soreness of some of the muscles of mastication.

When a plastic restoration is placed, not only must intercuspal occlusion be correct but prematurities must be eliminated in lateral and protrusive movements.

When a tooth is being prepared for an extracoronal restoration, adequate occlusal clearance for the required thickness of restoration in lateral and protrusive movements must be checked. Jaw movements should be reproduced as accurately as possible on an articulator in the laboratory, so that the restoration is constructed in harmony with functional jaw movements. When the restoration is placed on the tooth, jaw movements must be checked to ensure that premature contacts do not exist.

If a patient develops symptoms of muscle pain following insertion of a restoration, it should be examined for a prematurity in functional movements; on a metallic restoration this is usually revealed as a marked wear facet. Any prematurity should be removed without affecting intercuspal occlusal contacts. Symptoms disappear following removal of the occlusal interference.

UNDERCONTOURED RESTORATION

In an attempt to prevent premature occlusal contacts, some operators may go to the opposite extreme and fail to achieve any occlusal contact on the restoration. Where the restoration is large, the tooth may cease to have stable occlusal contacts and as a result over-erupt. This may increase the likelihood of food being packed between the teeth by plunger cusps. Also, premature contacts in lateral movements may develop later.

This type of error must be prevented by restoring teeth into correct and stable occlusion (Fig. 16.23). In the case of the large restoration,

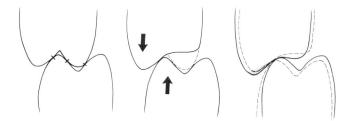

Fig. 16.23 *Left*: upper and lower teeth in stable occlusal contacts. *Middle*: the upper tooth has been restored into contact with the lower tooth but the occlusal contact is not stable, therefore overeruption can occur. *Right*: the teeth have moved from the positions indicated by an intermittent line to those indicated by a solid line; in lateral movements there is a premature contact which should be eliminated by removal of the shaded area.

reconstruction of the occlusal surface is more easily achieved in the laboratory with inlay wax than in the mouth with amalgam which is setting hard and to which additions cannot be made.

16.11 Electrosurgery

The removal of excess gingival tissue which has grown into a cavity may be achieved with electrosurgery. This technique has the advantage of causing minimal postoperative bleeding, which allows subsequent restoration of the tooth or impression taking.

The use of electrosurgery for cutting tissue was described early in this century, but its recent popularity has occurred because of the ready availability of inexpensive reliable electronic circuits for the production of fully rectified, filtered, high frequency current.

The cutting electrode is a thin wire (Fig. 16.24) which, when activated, passes through tissue like a knife through butter. In the tissue just in front of the wire, high frequency electrical energy jumps the gap to cause tissue destruction on a very limited scale. Provided that the

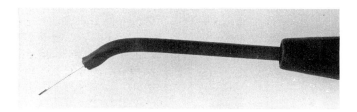

Fig. 16.24 The cutting electrode for electrosurgery is a thin wire.

electrode moves rapidly through the tissue, no lateral destruction of tissue occurs. The tissue heals as well as that cut with a scalpel, and considerably better than tissue that has been burnt by electrocautery. If the electrode is moved too slowly, severe tissue damage may occur; therefore, it should not be used by an inexperienced operator.

The tissue to be removed should be anaesthetized and the patient should lie on or hold the ground electrode. No metal instrument or denture should be present in the mouth, to prevent tissue burns, and the DSA should use a non-metallic large bore aspirator for the removal of offensive odour. The part of the mouth should be dried and the cutting electrode held by the operator over the tissue. Current is activated by the footswitch and the tissue should be cut cleanly and swiftly with the electrode. The power setting on the control unit is normally used at a midpoint setting; the current should be reduced if sparking occurs and increased if cutting is inadequate. Between strokes, the electrode should be cleaned with gauze soaked in 70% alcohol to maintain cutting efficiency; no current must be allowed to flow while the electrode is being cleaned. During cutting, contact of the electrode with metallic restorations should be avoided, to prevent pulpal damage which can occur on prolonged exposure. The excised excess tissue can normally be lifted away with an excavator.

After use, the cutting electrode should be cleaned in an ultrasonic bath prior to sterilization.

Electrosurgical equipment should not be used on or near people fitted with cardiac pacemakers, to prevent ventricular fibrillation which could be fatal.

When a large ball electrode is used, hypertrophic tissue can be removed by electrocoagulation in which heat is produced. Healing is less rapid.

Further details of electrosurgery will be found in a suitable text (Malone, 1974).

16.12 Failure of restorations

Many textbooks create the impression that restorations last for ever. However, this is not the case; indeed, a study in Scotland in 1983 showed that 50% of amalgam restorations failed within 5 years (Elderton, 1983). This is typical for restorations placed in general dental practice, but when the restorations have been placed by a single careful operator, a half-life of 10 years was found (Robinson, 1971).

Many failures can be attributed to poor technique and therefore the possible causes of failure will be considered in an attempt to make the operator more critical of the way he performs his own work. In view of the short life of restorations, it is advisable to leave in place restorations that are slightly less than perfect and review their status again in 6 months or a year. A balance must be struck between leaving a restoration with a chipped margin unassociated with caries and, on the other hand, a restoration with active caries at the margin.

INCORRECT PREPARATION OF THE TOOTH

1 Caries remaining at a margin or amelo-dentinal junction at the time of restoration may appear as 'recurrent' caries subsequently.
2 Enamel margins may be incorrectly finished for the restorative material; amalgam would chip when placed against a bevelled margin.
3 The preparation may be too shallow; a cast restoration could lack retention or amalgam fracture.
4 The preparation may have inadequate retentive form; the restoration would become dislodged.
5 There may be a failure to protect weakened cusps, which could fracture.

INCORRECT CHOICE OF RESTORATIVE MATERIAL

1 The material has insufficient strength for the chosen site.
2 The material displays excessive wear.

INCORRECT MANIPULATION OF MATERIAL

1 The material has not been mixed according to manufacturer's directions.
2 The material has not been completely packed into the cavity.
3 The material has been contaminated by moisture during insertion.
4 The material has been improperly contoured causing a gingival overhang, occlusal prematurity or defective approximal contact.

FAILURE OF THE MATERIAL

1 A cement restoration or lute of a cast restoration may dissolve.
2 Metals may corrode.
3 Tooth-coloured materials may discolour.

FAILURES NOT ATTRIBUTABLE TO THE RESTORATION

1 Caries on the same or another tooth surface may necessitate replacement of the restoration; this is particularly so in young patients where approximal caries leads to replacement of occlusal restorations.

2 Pulp disease may require removal of the restoration to reach the pulp.

3 The tooth may be extracted for another reason.

Bibliography

Bishop P. T. (1983) Frequency of accidental intravascular injection of local anaesthetics in children. *British Dental Journal*, **154**, 76–77.

British Dental Association (1991) *The Control of Cross infection in Dentistry*. British Dental Association, London.

Cawson R. A., Curson I. & Whittington D. R. (1983) The hazards of dental local anaesthetics. *British Dental Journal*, **154**, 253–258.

Elderton R. J. (1971) A modern approach to the use of rubber dam. *Dental Practitioner*, **21**, 187–193, 226–232, 267–273.

Elderton R. J. (1983) Longitudinal study of dental treatment in the general dental service in Scotland. *British Dental Journal*, **155**, 91–96.

Hill C. M. & Morris P. J. (1983) *General Anaesthesia and Sedation in Dentistry*. Wright, Bristol.

Howe G. L. & Whitehead F. I. H. (1981) *Local Anaesthesia in Dentistry*. Wright, Bristol.

Krejci R. F., Reinhardt R. A., Wentz F. M., Hardt A. B. & Shaw D. H. (1982) Effects of electrosurgery on dog pulps under cervical metallic restorations. *Oral Surgery, Oral Medicine and Oral Pathology*, **54**, 575–582.

Leon A. R. (1976) Amalgam restorations and periodontal disease. *British Dental Journal*, **140**, 377–382.

Lindhe J. (1984) *Textbook of Clinical Periodontology*. Munksgaard, Copenhagen.

Malone W. F. (1974) *Electrosurgery in Dentistry. Theory and Application in Clinical Practice*. Thomas, Springfield, Illinois.

Paul E. (1972) *A Practical Guide to Assisted Operating*. British Dental Association, London.

Robinson A. D. (1971) The life of a filling. *British Dental Journal*, **130**, 206–208.

Scully C. & Cawson R. A. (1982) *Medical Problems in Dentistry*. Wright, Bristol.

Smith N. J. D. (1980) *Dental Radiography*. Blackwell Scientific Publications, Oxford.

Thomson H. (1990) *Occlusion*, 2nd edn. Wright, London.

Torafson T., Kiger R., Selvig K. A. & Egelberg J. (1979) Clinical improvement of gingival conditions following ultrasonic versus hand instrumentation of periodontal pockets. *Journal of Clinical Periodontology*, **65**, 165–176.

Wise M. D. (1982) *Occlusion and Restorative Dentistry for the General Practitioner*. British Dental Association, London.

Index